Deep Core Healing

By Sharon Milne Barbour

Deep Core Healing

Contents

An Introduction to Deep Core Healing

Deep Core Healing is a transformational journey of accepting, releasing, and evolving beyond the emotional and energetic imprints that have created illness, imbalance, and pain within the human body and mind. It is a process that may begin with traditional clinical medicine while gradually integrating holistic healing, until eventually the individual becomes able to maintain ongoing wellness through energetic and spiritual alignment.

For Deep Core Healing to unfold, the human must hold a **pure intention to heal**. Once this intention is activated, the spiritual journey naturally expands, and the individual begins to evolve into a higher state of physical, emotional, and higher self soul plan awareness. This process has many layers, and a deeper understanding of spiritual knowledge is required to achieve lasting transformation.

Deep Core Healing addresses the negative energies stored within both the physical body and the ethereal light energy system. Throughout a human life, experiences are gathered, some beautiful and uplifting, others traumatic. Even when a person believes they have healed, emotional residue often remains deep within the core layers of the ethereal self. The ethereal light body is connected to the universal quantum domains creative intelligence which is connected to every ethereal and human physical cell, these unresolved energies continue to influence health, emotions, and life expression until released.

Clearing this deep core energy is essential for humanity's survival and evolution, and I know that this book will help you begin that process.

This book has been channelled through the Celestial Guardians of Earth, an alliance of ancient universal beings working alongside the overseers of the cosmos to assist humanity in its next stage of ascension. Within these pages, they will guide you through many forms of spiritual and human healing, as understood from the third-dimensional Earth perspective. They will also share examples of human life patterns, showing how spiritual evolution and Earth experience weave together across a lifetime. It is through this understanding that you will gain the tools for Deep Core Healing.

The Celestial Guardians are beings of high ascension, each holding ages of wisdom and compassion. They strive for harmony among universal challenges through unconditional love, standing beside humanity even through periods of self-destruction and collective darkness. Their quantum light works to dismantle the barriers that have shaped humanity over centuries and to restore remembrance of a more evolved and sacred way of being.

It is now the time to share this knowledge more openly, to help you move toward the higher ascension stages of your Earth journey. Every human is unique and will heal at different times, in different ways, and at different levels of ascension. No two paths are the same. Each human form arrives with a ethereal human essence, higher self, soul plan, celestial guides, and a lifelong Unison Guide who works in partnership with the Celestial Guardians to support the human mission chosen before Ethereal Earth connection. These celestial guides embrace the essence of each individual and unify the energies required to fulfil that mission for the greater good.

However, in recent human history, the global mission began to falter. And so, the awakening was initiated.

Humanity now moves through a collective shift marked by illness, war, environmental imbalance, and displacement. This global awakening was designed as a powerful moment of reflection a *"Stop and look"* phase calling humanity to change how it lives, treats one another, and honours Mother Earth.

Yet hope is rising. The balance is shifting as compassion, empathy, unity, and love begin to flood Earth's dimensional layers. For humanity to step into this higher frequency, each person must acknowledge responsibility for their own thoughts, behaviours, and actions. Healing must begin at the emotional core, moving through layers of energetic release and transformation.

Throughout your lifetime, you will move through phases of healing, learning, and spiritual growth depending on the lessons your ethereal light body and higher self have chosen and the contribution you are here to make to Earth's ascension. Deep Core Healing is one of the highest phases of this journey, empowering human individuals to step into the new developing Earth time line and become healers of humanity and Earth. Those who reach this phase will recognise the Celestial Guardians as allies, mentors, and companions on their spiritual path.

As humanity learns to work together, heart-to-heart, human-to-celestial guide, soul plan-to-quantum universe, the old layers of doubt dissolve and are replaced with trust. When this happens, the treasure chest of ancient knowledge and clarity opens, enabling the Earth human to rise into higher understanding and co-creation of the new ascension frequency.

This book provides the teachings, insights, and meditations required for this journey into Deep Core Healing. Your celestial guides walk beside you throughout this transformation. Set your intention with a pure heart, ask for guidance, healing, and love and you will begin to see the emergence of a new you...

...The true YOU.

Humanity is at a Turning Point

Humanity is experiencing a profound evolutionary shift in consciousness. This change is not random or accidental. It is part of a larger universal quantum plan designed to guide Earth and its people into a higher state of awareness, peace, and spiritual awakening.

For thousands of years, humanity has lived largely in a fear-based dimensional reality, focused on physical survival, linear thinking, and separation. But we are now stepping into a new **Quantum Era**, an age in which humanity is learning to exist as awakened multi-dimensional beings connected to higher intelligence and guidance and the collective human ascension path.

This transition will move humanity from a world of external authority to one of internal mastery and spiritual remembrance.

The Catalysts of Change

Global events in recent years such as Covid 19 acted as a catalyst to:

- Slow humanity down

- Interrupt unconscious living

- Break old patterns and systems

- Push individuals into self-reflection

- Open spiritual sensitivity

- Encourage re-evaluation of priorities

Many people experienced emotional upheaval, loss, uncertainty, or internal breakdowns, not as punishment, but as the beginning of a deep soul plan reset.

Humanity could not continue on the old Earth time line. The shift had to begin.

The Collective Awakening

This awakening is happening at every level:

- Physical

- Emotional

- Mental

- Spiritual

- Energetic

- Ethereal

- Quantum

As humans awaken, they begin to:

- Sense their celestial guides more clearly

- Question the nature of their reality

- Feel energy and frequency changes physically and around them

- Recognise their ethereal human essence and soul plan memories

- Witness synchronicities

- Develop greater intuition

- Learn to heal on a deeper level

This is the rise of Deep Core Healing, healing the stored emotional memory, karmic imprint, trauma, belief systems, and unconscious programming within the physical human and ethereal light bodies.

Healing is Personal and Collective

Every time one human heals:

- Their vibration rises

- Their frequency strengthens

- Their consciousness expands

- The Earth's collective energy grid becomes lighter

Human evolution is not only about survival or intelligence, but also about remembering who we truly are: Remember you are Eternal multi-dimensional ethereal light essences experiencing a physical human life for the purpose of Earth's evolution.

Your personal healing is not just for you; it contributes to humanity's ascension.

Guided by Universal Support

Humanity has never been alone in this process. Higher beings, often known as:

- Light Councils

- Intergalactic Councils

- Ascension Teams

- Celestial guides

- Higher self Support

- Humanity's Earth celestial guides - that have been assisting Earth for a millennia.

Their role is not to interfere but to guide, strengthen, illuminate, and support humanity in stepping into its higher potential. Many higher celestial guides telepathically connect to a physical human form on Earth, some guide telepathically, and others work through energetic frequency exchange.

As humanity rises in consciousness, we are learning to expand beyond traditional forms of communication and connection. We are rediscovering how to:

- Consciously recognise and identify our celestial guides

- Sense and understand their unique energetic signatures

- Receive communication through frequency rather than spoken language

- Trust the voice of higher intuition

- Develop telepathic receptivity

These abilities are not new; they are ancient human capacities being reawakened as we evolve into quantum-level awareness. As the collective ascends, these skills will become increasingly natural and effortless for many.

Our celestial guides are supporting this transition by transmitting knowledge through trance communicators, channels, and writers of higher wisdom, ensuring that humanity has access to the teachings required for the next phase of evolution.

Deep Core Healing – Why Now?

Humanity has reached a stage where:

- Emotional wounds

- Ancestral trauma

- Karmic agreements

- Past-life imprints

- Subconscious programming

can no longer remain buried.

For humanity to evolve into a higher dimension of unity and spiritual consciousness, these layers must be cleared from:

- The physical body

- The emotional body

- The mental body

- The ethereal light energy quantum field

- The soul plan imprint

This is the purpose of Deep Core Healing and the work you are now beginning.

Chapter one

Understanding the Journey of Change for Humanity

To help you start this journey of change I wish to share knowledge with you starting with the wakening of humanity.

Earth is in the process of an awakening unlike any other humanity has ever experienced on Earth. When a civilisation struggles to reach its full potential because its people cannot work in separation and not unity, it will eventually self-destruct, taking the life force space of the people with it.

Many millennia of humanity's history lie wasted and forgotten in the layers of Earth's dust. Many times, over our planet's history, civilisations have been rebuilt in the hope humanity can live as one. Always, there is the continued hope that a new world will emerge and exist in the continuous light energy of love and not the darkness of hate, doubt, and fear.

Earth's story is told across many of the universe's civilisations, used as a teaching example for others to learn from. It brings to them the lesson that if you do not listen to your life force space and respect your own kind, the utopia that is often sought is never found.

This awakening event that started in December 2019 onwards has lots of theories created by humans to explain what is happening to the world around you. But the simple fact is the overseers of *the universal quantum domains creative intelligence* (some see as the God source) and many high level ascensions celestial beings triggered this event. Humanity has been influenced by celestial beings for thousands of years and still is. These celestial beings vary from physical form to ethereal light transitional multi-dimensional beings. For the human language, the word experiment has been used for your understanding. There has been experiments over Earth's timeline creating humans and influencing them in various ways to try to create a sustainable high ascension of existence. One of these was for Earth to be part of the universal Ethereal Connection programme (some understand as incarnation) allowing many celestial beings to experience life on Earth as it struggles to ascend - setting themselves lessons to learn from this connection in a heavier energy existence. All of this knowledge was bought back to the *universal quantum domains knowledge pot*, to help them make our overseers make decisions about humanities future.

Our Earth has had celestial being visitors for millions of years, but a lot of evidence has not survived. The influence of these past ascension beings on Earth was mixed, as not all worked in the light. A long time ago, the overseers of the universe created the Light and Intergalactic Councils to pull together all the ascension beings working in the light energy for the highest good of all. With their telepathic skills and technology, they sought to bring their light across the universe, helping others to ascend into the light and love way of existing and Earth was chosen for this purpose.

Now go back over 12,000 years in Earth's history, when humans were starting to record the celestial beings on cave walls and gods and deities were created from their influence. Religions were sparked from the feeling of a force unseen, felt in the human heart from ethereal light essence source connected with the physical human's body. This force is what you understand as the God energy.

Think of these celestial beings in the light as friends of humanity. Humans have free will to a point; there were gaps in the overseers' influence when they left humanity alone and as Earth's history shows darkness came, and with that, wars. So, at various times when humanity needed a push back into the light, they telepathically influenced our minds, trying to guide humanity onto the path of ascension again. This ascension path helps humans to be influenced to love each other, bringing kindness to humanity and the Mother Earth. Our celestial guides know humans are cable of ascension where they could heal themselves and with their minds and nature, if they reached the four to five-dimensional clarity of understanding.

At the end of Earth's second world war, the overseers felt they were failing humanity and Mother Earth, so they called upon many celestial beings from the light across the universe to come and help them. They became observers, ethereally connected to human beings, and celestial guides. Through the higher self and soul plan many celestial beings set missions to help Earth ascend, they stopped just gathering information and learning lessons for their own ascension path and worked to help humanity and the Earth survive.

Through these new alliances, they influenced technology, and the progression of humanity and one of their missions was the hope humanity would develop clean energy and have a global unity with no more wars, just peace. Clean technology does exist on Earth, but it does not feed the greed of the rich; as it should be free to all, but it remains at this time hidden from the Earth societies by the power over darker energies. The overseers sometimes had to accept these darker influences were more powerful and they were with it affecting the light forces influence on Earth. They always hoped the humans would be strong enough to eradicate this on their own with an ethereal human essence, higher self soul plan, celestial guides, and higher self connection support group network.

The overseers brought their message through celestial ascension beings to Earth's governments through physical interaction and mind connection, but this stayed behind closed doors and was misused by those who had the privilege of meeting these beings. The overseers then decided to bring the message of change to humans through trance communicators, channelers and holistic healers placed that had agreed within their soul plan to spread their purpose of quantum light and new hope into humanity. This would have to be done in the awakening period on Earth.

The overseers then had to plan a strategy to build on this progress. They needed to slow the world down and give humans time to reflect and support each other in times of crisis, to create a situation that would influence the minds of the scientists and leaders to talk to each other. Also for hidden agendas to be revealed to the public domain of human society, so humanity could question their reality. This was also a time for all spiritual people to start using their telepathic mind power links to send for example remote healing, so they understood the power of telepathic connection. But the main reason was to help heal Mother Earth so she and humanity could survive.

This chosen virus infection is no worse than anything else that had yet been created on Earth but was designed to open minds rather than destroy humanity. As with any illness it would take the weak of physical body, and it had the hidden facet of also taking the strong, this had to be placed in their consciousness in their DNA, to be triggered when the virus struck, and this was to bring the fear base around this virus.

As the virus took hold round the Earth the overseers could see the shift in humanity's thinking and many things were being revealed to them through changes being imposed on the population. Money was not as important, materialistic items could be lived without, and what they had was valued more. Families were divided due to quarantine restrictions, and this has helped humanity appreciate each other and the freedom they once had. This period of time has unleashed pent up anger, for example over how humanity treated each other because of the colour of their skins. These changes need to be bought to the surface to shift the old energy to the new high Earth frequency, it has bought unrest for many but also created positive change. Also relationships have been tested and revealed weakness bringing change. People have started to question how they live and are being drawn to the smaller community concept. In the lock down period images emerged of Mother Earth healing, seas clearing, animals coming back to old habitats, because humans have not been actively trampling the Earth, and this meant less pollution.

The overseers observed firstly those humans that had to isolate in their dwellings, were finding solitude, solidarity, and the challenge of mind and self-awakening through this process. Secondly, those humans who were named as being on the front line, which were the key workers and the sick. These humans found challenges of mind and body, solidarity, some solitude, new inner strength and self-awakening. No matter their religion or creed they had to dig deep inside to find strength to get through this time period of change.

Many humans have experienced isolation and loneliness at the end of their lives, but their soul plan level was always prepared and supported during this process and the higher self and chosen celestial guides kept the ethereal human essence safe on its transition home. Humans that were already awakened have used the awakening time line to rediscover themselves and their true ordained Earth's path. They had to dig deeper than they ever had before to reconnect to the quantum universal energy and reach their soul plan level and life's purpose. This was achieved though further healing processes. They are learning about trusting their intuition, which comes from the soul plan level of the human experience.

It has been observed that many humans cannot understand this virus, as the number ill and dying were lower than that, say, of a bad flu epidemic. All sorts of conspiracy theories were circulated, being fed by the darker three-dimensional fear-based energies. It does not matter if this was a human built contagion, or Earth's biological reaction to technology and pollution, it was triggered by an ordained off world higher power source to try and help humanity. The decision was made on this Earth's time line based on previous Earth events that led to this point of desperation. The overseers and Intergalactic Council had really hoped it would not come to this but stepped into bring a needed awakening to humanity, so to give Mother Earth a chance to heal and reset her energies.

Many celestial beings working in the light have been a huge part of this awakening period, and they have bought new celestial guides to every light worker channeller. The purpose of these celestial guides is to help channel the light to Earth and one way of this is through telepathic communication and channelling. They are the architects of a new light program the **'Quantum Era'** to help humanity. Many light workers who have been on the path for a few of our Earth years, are now merging with other light workers energies to work together. These are higher self's and ethereal human essences that have been part of ancient times plans and have gained great knowledge and are known to some as Avatars essences. Example of these ancient ethereal light essences include the founders of major world religions, such as Jesus, Buddha, and Krishna. An Avatar is born not to show us how great they are, but to give us hope that humanity can gain a state of high consciousness that the avatar human has attained.

This ancient knowledge is now going to emerge through teachings that are being downloaded to a chosen few leading light workers as the awakening unfolds on Earth. These humans are predestined for this knowledge, and they have high ascended twelve celestial guides working with them. Some of our celestial guides work within the twelve essences, as within it, it creates imagination, effective communication, tolerance, self-sufficiency, self-determination, cooperation, optimism, and dynamism exists. Virtually everything the number twelve does is expressed creatively. Twelve is the base of creation of the universe and the creative mind. Twelve is used to create what is needed in all sorts of existence in creation.

For your understanding they are working in unities of twelve that symbolises the power of the universe overseers, this can be found in Earth's history, reflected in the era of Jesus New Testament of the Bible, such as Jesus' selection of twelve apostles, he said, *"That choice was deliberate, with each apostle representing one of the twelve tribes of Israel"* and don't forget the twelve cities in Atlantis and their twelve guardian celestial beings the 'Rays'. There are twelve main gods in Greek mythology, Odin had twelve sons in Norse mythology, twelve disciples of Christ in Christianity, and twelve Imams in the Islam religion. The samples I have given might seem male energy driven but through history disciples and light leaders have been of mixed gender trying to spread the light. In modern day society at the moment the divine female energy is more at the fore front as leaders of the light. This varies depending on the Earth's energies of the time, but our celestial guides are now working to bring the more masculine energies into balance the high frequency energies again. In the most of cases number twelve is actually a representation of authority and perfection.

If you are one of these chosen leaders of twelve, you will have twelve disciples, this could be people in your teaching groups, mentoring or a friend/family member you are guiding on their spiritual path. These leaders will be the light of twelve beings on Earth guiding them. Some of the twelve group with them, then become leading teachers themselves, who will then be sent twelve disciples to guide. This will create a ripple effect out through Earth's consciousness. The higher self of the twelve will always stay soul plan linked even if the destined Earth life drifts them apart.

When you are part of a group of twelve on Earth, your higher self stays linked when part of that Earth circle of twelve. They meet off world in a high dimensional space of unison energy. Higher self's come from various sources of creation and can be multi-dimensional transitional forms to physical presence. So, the space of unison energy allows all to exist and communicate in the circle with the leader of light in the centre. As this circle on Earth grows and the individuals develop, some will become teachers on Earth. This will lead them to become a leader of light of twelve further humans creating another circle. The higher selves in the unison energy, can be part of their own development circle, and multi-task being a leader of light for a new circle. Highly ascended higher self's have the ability to be in several places at once giving their teachings to others. All leaders of light would have had an ethereal connection to an Earth physical human form to help them work with and understand human individuals. As they ascend on Earth in the dimensional energies, their higher self grows as well. The higher self can become an ascended master leader of light, that runs many circles in the unison energy off world, as well as overseeing their Earth life. The unison space circles of twelve are forever growing and ascending causing the ripple effect of growth and ascension for humanity on Earth.

Those that are the leaders of spiritual knowledge such as light workers like light worker channellers or holistic healers will experience great energy shifts at this time, and they will be asked to be light channelers of spiritual knowledge. This will create a different perception for them and their communication with the celestial guides will be on a higher vibration. Their new mission with this ascension is to help humanity heal, and this will be done through these channelled light reading messages, which will involve energy healing and guidance messages. These light worker channellers will hold the light our celestial guides are channelling to Earth, guiding others to understand this new light energy, and spread their teachings. For the humans with this mission to achieve their full potential they will need to go through the Deep Core Healing.

Chapter two

Understanding your Celestial Guides and Their Terminology

You might wonder and question who the celestial beings are I will mention for your knowledge. So I will lay out before you this knowledge and terminology they have created with the human language. Our celestial guides are part of this Deep Core Healing journey and is for you as individuals, but also for the sake of the human collective to understand them.

The Quantum universe is overseen by a high ascension light beings called the overseers. These beings of pure light consciousness exist in the universe's high energy dimensional levels, overseeing all quantum source creation in the universe, including our Earth. These celestial beings using the Quantum domains energy can manifest and create miracles of creation as well as destroying them. Humanity has tried to understand this for a long time and see these actions as miracles. This has led humanity to worship the unseen forces of wonder in the universe, creating the three-dimensional understanding of this as the GOD energy.

The overseers of the universe create galaxies, planets, and life where they think it will thrive for the greater good of the universe. They work tirelessly, creating a balance of all energies, masculine, feminine, light, and dark, trying to give all ascension life a chance to thrive. Ascension life is all life that can evolve, with intelligence to one day ascend way beyond their first capabilities of that first spark of quantum life.

The overseers create life on planets trying to create a balanced utopia. An example of the overseers' work is when they took the molten volcanic rock world known as Earth and slowly populated her with life, adjusting the planet's environment over billions of Earth years. Life on Earth came from other high vibrational planets with the aim to create similar worlds. Not all things go to plan though. For example, asteroids hitting Earth brought new bacteria and disease to Earth, and destruction from shifts of the planet's crust and polar axis over millions of years. As you can imagine these natural types of events quite often upset the plans for these developing planets, but yet all add to the experiment of existence. An example of this is the Planet Mars in our solar system. Mars was eventually left to naturally die and the overseers put their energy into evolving Earth.

Each time there was a natural extinction event on Earth, the overseers had a choice to continue with the Earth experiment by restarting Earth's eco system with new species or letting it evolve naturally. Over time they did a mixture of this, adding new life then letting Earth evolve naturally from that point. Then around three hundred thousand years ago, when Earth had reached a pure energy level again for highly ascended human life, they intervened again, and this was known as the period of the Atlantis experiments. *(You can find out about the Atlantis Earth period in my channelled book 'The Light within Atlantis').*

A long, long time ago the overseers got to the point where

they needed help to fulfil their works of creation in the universe. This was mainly to help monitor galaxies and planets by creating a universal knowledge pot of information to help with future decisions. They felt the species that had evolved to a highly intelligent state of being, could be given some responsibility to take their own knowledge and help other planets and celestial beings. They reached out to all the high ascending celestial beings of creation working in the light energy of unconditional love. From them they created councils made up of many ascended celestial beings from throughout the universe.

Light Councils

One of the first councils formed was called the Light Council, made up of various celestial beings that would collectively oversee the galaxies, with each galaxy having its own Light Council. They are either physical or light beings in high multi-dimensional transitional energy with the mission of being architects of evolution in the universe. They also take the step to help planets and individual celestial beings of all ascension levels by channelling their knowledge to them. But they do not ethereally connect to a physical being existence like an Earth human. Each Light Council has twelve members, and they have a member that is linked to each dimensional layer of the universe. This is so the balance of all is always monitored.

These beings are called the **'Ray'** recognised by their frequency and the divine chosen energy and teachings they each bring with them. They resonate on such a high pure love frequency that lower energy beings will see them as bright light forms, with each varying in colour depending on their frequency vibration and purpose. To the human eye they are interpreted as bright light with wispy bits of energy as they move. To you the energy might look like wings that pulsate behind them as they vibrate their amazing frequency with light, harmonic sound, and colour vibration. They communicate mind to mind in the light, colour vibration and harmonic sound frequency, in the desired language that is required. They have the ascension level to be in thousands of places and minds at once, always giving and receiving whatever is needed for the species they are helping.

They carefully select those to whom they choose to reveal themselves, generally choosing beings on a high ascension path; in Earth's case they are called light workers. These 'Ray' beings are connected to the divine quantum source of the overseers in the twelfth dimension and beyond.

Earth's Milky Way galaxy has a Light Council with twelve of these light beings and they have been working with us on a daily basis over the last 300,000 years. They work in unison with the dimensional layers one to twelve and I will now reveal them to you.

Dimensions

Dimension is a word given to humanity by our celestial guides to help us understand the layers of energy of existence in the universe. The dimensions I explain to you are linked to the universal quantum domain creative energy of intelligence. Laid out in this section is the celestial guides translation for your understanding that was channelled for the Earth book *'A Journey through Creation'*. I have heard some say there is not any dimensions, but there are many forms of existence and we all need to try to understand this in our human language and 3D reality. Imagine a sack that had 12 various layers of objects from Earth, at the bottom is a layer of rocks presenting the first dimension, the heaviest energy layer. Then the last layer twelfth dimension at the top of the sack is light feathers presenting the lightest purist energy layer of existence. If you throw the rocks into water they sink and the feathers float - get the picture.

A deeper understanding of these energies significantly contributes to spiritual development. Personally, it has enhanced my own healing and trance communication journey and deepened my connection with various celestial guides.

First Dimension (1D)

• Amber Ray is the guardian of the first dimension. This luminous being holds the responsibility of maintaining the energy balance on Earth and is intricately linked to the human Earth chakra and meridian points, which serves as your grounding connection to our home planet.

• Intricate layers of physical matter of planets are known as the first dimension (1D).

• Consciousness of physical matter creates the physical planets.

• Rock matter exhibits a response to sound and emits a subtle, low-level acoustic vibration reaction, suggesting a rudimentary form of intelligence.

• Chemical bonds continuously form and interact with one another, each responding at distinct frequencies to create the diverse array of rocks, crystals, and minerals.

• Rocks are made up of various compositions, then if another element was added it will adapt to it and evolve which shows intelligence. Rocks and crystals can retain a memory in energy form.

• This vibration, known as the first dimension level, connects with the energies of the second dimension (2D) and third dimension (3D) that exist above and within it.

• Within our planets 1D layers, you can uncover the remnants of ice ages, cataclysmic meteorite events, celestial phenomena, and the footprints of celestial being occupation. These imprints, etched over millennia's, are imprinted within the very fabric of 1D existence, evident in the crystal layers and rock formations on the Earth planet.

• Earth's water is part of the first dimension and supports various forms of life in the 2D and 3D dimensions.

• 1D showed a basic intelligence that 1D and 2D dimensions work together to support each other giving of invisible signals from inter-reacting with the universal quantum domains creative intelligence source.

Second Dimension (2D)

• In the second dimension level of existence on Earth, we encounter the consciousness of elemental vibration embodied by the light being known as Emerald Ray. This powerful being serves as a healer for organic physical life.

• The first and second dimensions produce the atmosphere of air and Earth elements in which organic plant life can thrive which helps sustain human life.

• In the 2D realm of existence on Earth, we encounter the consciousness of elemental vibration. Elemental beings exist in metaphysical level and help to look after 1D and 2D levels.

• Earth is home to a vast array of biodiversity in its flora and fauna. The planet boasts an incredible diversity of insects, mammals, and aquatic species that can communicate with each other through vibrational language and bio-chemical signals.

• Trees and plants are intelligent and communicate through its intricate root system and vibration. For instance, roots can detect drought conditions and signal the leaves to limit transpiration, thereby conserving water. Plants possess their own unique language, combining frequency, vibration, and chemicals to create a complex communication system for pollination and protection.

• The plants and oceans on Earth are the lungs of the Planet.

Third Dimension (3D)

• In Earth's third dimension (3D), we encounter the celestial being known as Fire Red Ray, who oversees this dimension.

Fire Red Ray plays a vital role in nurturing the warrior of sacred courage, fostering inner peace, and existing within the multi-dimensional layers of the galaxy's planets, including Earth.

• Humans are 3D celestial beings and struggling in our modern times to understand their universe. The revelation of quantum particles, with their mind-boggling properties, served as a catalyst for scientists to question the very fabric of reality.

• Simultaneously, those in the 3D reality embarking on a spiritual quest find themselves grappling with the profound mysteries of existence. Seeking to decipher the spiritual language that resonates within you all, they embark on a journey of self-discovery and enlightenment. Through introspection and contemplation, they strive to unlock the secrets of the ethereal human essence, forging a deeper connection with themselves and the world around them.

• Earth humans have celestial guides and a higher self soul connection.

• The ethereal body also known as the quantum body, is a concept that encompasses the energy field responsible for holding the physical form together in the 3D reality.

• Earth humans are aware of their five senses, but there exists a sixth sense, an inner knowing that eludes visual perception. This connection originates from a higher self level of the soul plan connection, intricately linked to human sub-consciousness. When nurtured, this connection allows us to tap into the higher dimensions and our quantum body and access the creative intelligence of the universe. In the Earth realm third dimension existence, such contemplation rarely occupies our day-to-day thoughts. Instead, you can find yourself engrossed in the task of constructing your own third dimension reality, a process that can overwhelm many, leading to physical and mental ailments.

• In the 3D levels Earth humans can learn to self-heal. A well-functioning human body possesses a clear and uninterrupted flow of energy from the universal quantum domain source. When a human being falls ill, it is not the fault of the universal quantum domain, but rather a result of the human individual's own actions. Living in a challenging reality often leads to stress and anxiety, which accumulate as heavy energy within the body, subsequently obstructing the natural flow of life-giving energy from creation.

• Earth humans' perception of reality is limited to our busy daily connections we make in our third dimension world. However, when we take a moment to still our minds, the vibrations within our bodies undergo a positive transformation. This allows our physical body and mind to elevate to a higher level of fourth to fifth dimension energy, enabling you to connect with your ethereal form and the quantum energies that created you. The convergence of human science and spirituality is ushering in a new 'Quantum Era' of human evolution on Earth. As human science and spirituality converge, maintaining a state of calmness becomes crucial to allow the quantum creative intelligence to operate effectively.

• Earth humans find solace within the safety of their 3D cocoon, believing that they have a firm grasp on their identity and reality. But at their soul plan level, sub-conscious and DNA is questions that need to be answered. They need to discover who they truly are, but the world in which they reside is fraught with numerous of threats. It is through the path of ascension and evolution that they will unravel the depths of their true self and manifest a reality that humanity has long yearned for – a reality that is secure and nurturing.

• Earth is a diverse world of unique cultures from nomad Amazon tribes to city dwellers and many religions and belief systems. There is love, compassion kindness, fear, hate and self-doubt. Most of the Earth cultures are run around money and materialistic values, this sadly stops the environmental green energy that is needed to help save the Mother Earth. The main thing is humanity is not learning from past mistakes and only when they do this can they ascend.

Fourth Dimension (4D)

At the fourth dimension level, we encounter the consciousness of transition and the light being known as the Violet Ray. This formidable entity serves as a guiding light, leading you away from negative energies such as karma, self-doubt, and despair. Instead, it offers you wisdom, love, transformation, and the ultimate truth, helping all Earth beings align with their ethereal connection and the soul and the higher self. This is the key to stepping out of the 3D reality and onto the 4D steppingstone energy bridge that leads to the fifth dimension.

• The fourth dimension is understood as the steppingstone to the fifth dimension. It serves as a gateway to a realm of higher energy, transcending the third dimension reality. There are three primary methods through which you can establish contact with the fourth dimension. The first method is through meditation, the second method involves entering the dream state, where connections with the human ethereal body and subconscious mind can enter a state of Astral travel to the fourth dimension. This is for knowledge, healing and communication with other celestial beings. The third method entails shifting your perspective find your true purpose and embracing spirituality. By finding and living your truth and aligning yourself with higher principles, you can elevate your ethereal energy and traverse the higher planes of existence. This transformation is facilitated by the practice of meditation, which serves as a guiding force in your spiritual journey.

• 4D is where ascending celestial beings start to enhance their telepathic connections and learn to self-heal. The fourth dimension serves as the gateway that allows celestial beings to physically manifest and establish telepathic connections with each other. They possess the ability to choose whether to remain unseen, operating at the fourth and fifth dimensional levels, often interacting with you through dreams, deep meditation, or trance-like states.

• This dimension is where celestial beings begin to release materialistic values, time restrictions, and embrace the significance of unity and collaboration for the greater good of all.

Fifth Dimension (5D)

• The fifth dimension, often referred to as the love dimension, is where all celestial beings begin to encounter the consciousness of unconditional love. This profound state of being is embodied by the light being known as Pink Ray. Pink Ray's primary purpose is to disseminate the energy of love throughout the Milky Way galaxy, with a special focus on assisting Earth's human inhabitants in cultivating self-awareness and fostering an open-hearted spirit of generosity through the guidance of unconditional love.

• Some Earth humans from the science concept see the 5D as a conceptual stage, unobservable micro dimension of space. But it is like the fourth dimension, the fifth dimension represents a realm beyond your current state of human consciousness. It is a space where the limitations of your minds and bodies can be transcended, allowing for a harmonious fusion of your physical form with the ethereal essence energy. This paves the way for a complete multi-dimensional transcendence, where humanity can progress beyond the fifth dimension and evolve to freely traverse the universe, learning to start shedding their physical form at will and reclaiming it when desired. The fifth dimension serves as a significant milestone on this transformative journey.

• When celestial beings in physical form ascend to the fifth dimension, they enter a state of super consciousness connected to the quantum domains pure creative intelligence, a higher level of awareness. In this state, you will be free from thoughts and emotions that weigh you down or hold you back. You will simply exist, fully present and conscious. You will have the ability to perceive and understand everything that defines the fifth dimension as a pure space of reality.

• The concept of time, as understood in our third dimension reality, will no longer dictate the actions of humanity.

• Elevated star children and light worker channellers are on Earth to help humanity ascend. When they access this 5D energy, they experience mental clarity. Light worker channellers can experience a sense of detachment from the 3D reality while delivering messages to the recipient, fully aware of the past over human essence. The more a light worker channeller operates within this 4D and 5D energy, the more they ascend as both physical and ethereal beings, growing stronger and more enlightened.

• New knowledge is constantly being discovered in the fields of science and spirituality, allowing Earth humans to gain a deeper understanding of the universe. By merging these two extremes, you can elevate your understanding and ultimately aid in the evolution of humanity to the fifth dimension.

• 5D physical beings participating in the ethereal connection program, such as Earth humans, individuals begin to transcend the need for a soul plan and higher self. This evolution occurs as they become capable of undergoing the ascension process necessary for progression. Guidance during this transformative journey is provided by the Intergalactic Council, as 5D celestial beings can participate in these councils.

Sixth Dimension (6D)

• Within this extraordinary sixth dimension, you will encounter the consciousness of creative ideas, personified by the celestial being of Yellow Ray. Its primary role is to guide celestial beings in controlling their emotions and discovering joy in their existence, even amidst the darker aspects of their emotional landscape. By freeing them from the grip of lower energies, this being empowers you to surpass your limitations and attain heightened spiritual awareness.

• It is worth mentioning that the 6D reality represents a purer space, serving as the initial stage where the physical body can transcend into an ethereal light form.

• Telepathic abilities are greatly enhanced in the sixth dimension. Physical celestial beings prioritise the well-being of their planets to ensure longevity for all inhabitants. Those who have ascended to this level also have access to universal knowledge from the quantum domain creative source of intelligence. However, they are guided by their Intergalactic Council on how to utilise resources for the benefit of their societies and the greater good of all.

• The 6D ascension process also enhances the planet, creatures, and flora, as well as altering the cellular structure of the celestial being's physical make up. This cellular enhancement can lead to self-healing though telepathic mind control over the body cellular structure. This enhancement also allows celestial beings to start manifesting objects and create a positive future.

• When celestial beings reach the 6D ascension stage they can be invited to join the 'Universal Ethereal Connection Program' this also applies to 7D to 10D celestial beings.

Seventh Dimension (7D) & Eighth Dimension (8D)

• **The seventh dimension (7D)** level is a door to the consciousness of harmonic sound over seen by light being Azure Ray. This light being brings the essence of comfort that gives strength to all celestial life with abundance of love. This harmonic frequency of energy brings compassion, empathy, non-judgemental thoughts, patience, kindness, forgiveness, gratitude, and sincerity. Once a celestial civilisation has a balance of these comforting energies, they will have clarity of mind and intelligence of the way forward.

• **The eighth dimension level (8D)** – is the consciousness of new creative manifestation over seen by light being Translucent Ray. This light being is the divine source teacher, leading the way that helps physical celestial beings such as humans stay true to the spiritual divine path. Translucent Ray brings knowledge to lower energy planet's atmosphere when the time is right for humans' further development to aid evolution. The required teachings are downloaded from the quantum universal knowledge library records to the being that connects with this source of new knowledge.

• Celestial beings in these two dimensions possess extraordinary abilities that allow them to teleport effortlessly across distances. They also have the power to manifest physical objects and structures, as well as manipulate and transport massive objects with the sheer force of their thoughts. As they advance from 7D to 8D, their powers are enhanced, but some species may encounter limitations in this progression. Additionally, some celestial beings may require technological assistance to fully utilise their abilities. Furthermore, the values associated with material possessions will shift within these dimensions.

• Physical celestial beings are taking on the forms of multi-dimensional transcendent beings that can transcend through the universe or through energy portals. The cellular structure change for this starts in 5D and 6D ascension process. This entails a transformation of their physical bodies into an ethereal form, allowing for the breakdown of their cellular structure and transcendence of the boundaries of existence. Their conscious minds maintained this ethereal state until they reached their intended destination, where they revert to their physical form. This extraordinary ability to surpass the limitations of the material world serves as a testament to their advanced spiritual evolution.

• In these two dimensions celestial beings also have very advanced technology for star ships, communications processes and creating spaces of unison for off world gatherings.

Ninth Dimension (9D)

• The overseer of the ninth dimension level (9D) is light being Astral Blue Ray - the consciousness of manifestation. This light being's purpose is to manifest the energy needed for, example, to oversee the incarnated souls, from selection until they return home to source. It also oversees the communication between the physical body, ethereal body, physical planet, and the celestial cosmos matrix. This is to ensure the psychic, intuitive gifts of telepathic and outer body teleportation can create the required reality between the celestial being and the quantum domain source, home planet or realm, their star system and the galaxy.

• Telepathic communication is enhanced with the ability for collective communication with groups of celestial beings. This does not involve reading each other's thoughts but rather interpreting diverse language foundations and comprehending each other without intrusion. A 9D energy pattern is created to facilitate this form of communication. Many species in 9D have long distant mind links and can help facilitate other beings to communicate long distant.

• 9D celestial beings can telepathically tune into the quantum domains creative intelligence for portal travel with the intention of their desired destination, and it will indicate whether a portal already exists for them to access. If not, the creative intelligence will determine if a new portal can be safely created and will document this information for future travellers. As celestial beings ascend through the dimensional layers of the universe, the ability to travel longer distances through multi-dimensional means becomes possible. When utilising these portals, individuals do not physically transport their solid form. Instead, they transmute into ethereal energy light beings held in suspension and then reform into physical beings upon reaching their destination. This process allows for safe and efficient travel across vast distances within the universe.

• Some celestial 9D species can seamlessly blend in with Earth's humanity by using telepathic mind control to appear humanoid to the population. This level of mind control allows them to walk among Earth humans undetected, showcasing their incredible abilities to adapt and integrate into different societies. They only do this if they are needed to aid the ascension of that civilisation for the greater good of all.

• Some celestial 9D species like the Arcturians have the remarkable ability to take on physical forms at levels up to 9D physical existence and manipulate their transition into the civilisation they are assimilating with.

• In the 9D existence, not all structures on 9D planets are permanent; they are manifested as needed.

• In 9D many celestial forms undergo a transformation, causing them to rely more on quantum energy sources for sustenance. This shift occurs as their physical form transcends into a more ethereal light source of being. Every cell in their body undergoes alterations during this evolutionary process, changing the need for food and liquid in take to stay alive.

Tenth Dimension (10D) & Eleventh Dimension (11D)

• **The tenth dimension level (10D)** represents the pinnacle of consciousness, revealing the ultimate truth and is overseen by the light being known as Indigo Ray. Indigo Ray serves as the gateway to knowledge, wisdom, and unravelling the mysteries of the universe dimensional layers through the realms of truth. Guiding numerous celestial civilisations,

Indigo Ray facilitates the healing of planetary energies. Indigo Ray celestial guides species in enhancing their planet's ley lines for healing and communication processes, as well as assisting all celestial beings in tapping into the quantum domain's creative intelligence for new knowledge to enhance their societies.

• **Eleventh dimension level (11D)** represents the second highest consciousness of the universe and is overseen by the light being known as Lilac Ray. Lilac Ray is the guardian of the twelve principal laws of the universe, guiding celestial beings in incorporating these truths into their teachings. By following these laws, celestial beings can achieve a harmonious balance in their spiritual and physical existence.

• Celestial beings at 10D are mainly consciousness, a collective of light beings. Beings from 3D to 9D physical and ethereal bodies operate in lower dimensional energy, making it not always possible for them to visually perceive the 10D to 12D realms. To provide an analogy, it is akin to Earth elemental beings who have elevated themselves to a metaphysical 4D existence, beyond the visible spectrum in the Earth plane. The reason why beings from 3D to 9D cannot physically see is because 10D exists in a higher dimension, beyond their current level of perception. Their physical and ethereal bodies operate in lower dimensional energy, making it impossible for them to always perceive the higher realms visually or telepathically.

• Some of the celestial beings that exist in these two dimensions are seen as highly ascended ethereal beings of love, for example often referred to Earth as Archangels. The celestial beings in these two dimensions have transcended their physical form, evolving into multi-dimensional transcendent light beings. Upon shedding all material possessions, their presence now exists solely for the greater good of the universe. The overseers of the universe create a realm of existence for them to form a collective and guide them on their continued ascension journey.

Twelfth Dimension (12D)

• Light being Silver Ray, oversees the twelfth dimension level (12D) - the consciousness of the quantum domain source. This light being emanates from the divine energy of creation, connecting everything through the silver ray of love that permeates everything in the universe and its twelve dimensions. Silver Ray collaborates closely with the other Rays and the overseers to ensure that the teachings of true compassion and love remain at the forefront of all interactions. Additionally, Silver Ray facilitates the reunion of twin souls on celestial planes, uniting them to work together for the greater good.

• In the twelfth dimension, we are introduced to the infinite and ever-expanding creative intelligence that encompasses all knowledge that has ever existed throughout the universe's lifespan. This concept is intricately linked back to the zero point in the quantum domain. Picture a perpetually expanding circle that ripples outwards, continuously reflecting back in on itself, creating layers of energy and intelligence. This phenomenon represents the quantum core of all existence. Within these layers of energy new galaxies, stars, unison collective space, planets, celestial beings, and creatures at levels 1D to 10D are constantly being created, while others collapse and bring an end to life. This cycle has been ongoing for billions of years.

• In 12D is where we find the overseers of the universe, they are a collective of beings all working as one. They exist beyond the understanding of the twelve-dimensional space. They are a part of everything in the universe and have a core connection from the first spark of the quantum domain to the infinitely expanding energy of the universe. They are overseers not only of this universe, but of others as well. They are the most highly ascended beings in existence and are the architects of our known universe. They ensure that new galaxies, solar systems, planets, and celestial beings are provided with the necessary energy for positive growth and outcomes. They learn from failure, continuously expanding their own knowledge, which in turn helps young universes that are being born to develop.

I hope this brief breakdown of each dimension helps guide your understanding of these dimensions and where your celestial guides come from. All life is interconnected through these dimensions, ultimately leading back to the universal quantum domain - the source of creative intelligence where all moments are held within multi-verse time lines in the infinite energy source. This inter-connectedness can be visualised as a circle of existence, where life is both born and ends, continuously creating and learning for eternity.

Intergalactic Councils

Intergalactic Councils oversee individual planets, and evolving life forms. Each Intergalactic Council has a Light Council member, aiding with the communication needed for success. The mission of the Intergalactic Councils is to bring all ascended beings they are ordained to help under one umbrella of guidance and protection. They guide all species to work together in unity, creating new alliances and guiding those selected along the ascension path of light. Each celestial species at this level of high ascension consciousness selects members of their own high councils to sit on the Intergalactic Council. Within the Intergalactic Council are smaller councils, one for each planet made up of the species that are in an alliance to oversee their chosen planet. They are the architects and keepers of Earth's history and knowledge, which is fed to the Intergalactic Council and the universal quantum source knowledge library.

Humanity's Celestial Guides

Throughout human history and across various cultures, people have spoken of unseen helpers - beings of light, wisdom, and compassion who watch over us and guide our Earth life journey. These celestial guides are also can be known as universal celestial guides, angels, or guardian spirits or guardian angels. Despite the different names, the underlying message remains the same: we are never alone. Beyond the physical 3D realm, there exists celestial physical and light beings and a benevolent intelligence that supports, protects, and gently celestial guides us towards growth, healing, and our spiritual purpose.

Celestial guides are higher-multi-dimensional light or physical beings who guide humanity. They are mainly free from ego and earthly attachments, operating from a place of unconditional love and divine wisdom. These celestial guides offer guidance through intuition, dreams, synchronicities, signs, and inner knowing. Some may appear as protectors in times of danger, while others may impart knowledge and truths in moments of stillness. Many celestial guides work behind the scenes, orchestrating events of our soul plans for our highest good.

What humans call Angels, for example, are often seen as messengers carrying divine energy and insight. Guardian angels are believed to be assigned to us at birth, accompanying us throughout our lives and providing silent support during times of hardship, celebration, and transformation. All celestial guides may include ancestral ethereal essences, ascended masters, or cosmic beings aligned with the soul plan's greater purpose. While they respect our free will, they gently guide us towards our soul plans journey, hoping that we will listen and be receptive to their presence when we ask for help.

For humanity, the universal celestial guides represent more than just spiritual assistance - they serve as powerful symbols of the interconnectedness between the material and ethereal spiritual realms. In a world often plagued by fear, grief, and uncertainty, these celestial guides embody hope, higher truth, and the unseen love that envelops us.

They inspire us to trust our inner voice, follow our soul plans path, and remember that we are spiritual beings having a human experience, not the other way around.

Connecting with these celestial guides does not require elaborate rituals. A sincere heart, a quiet space, and an open mind are all that is needed. Whether through prayer, meditation, channelling, journalling, or simply asking for signs, the key is a simple invitation: *"Show me the way. Walk beside me today."* Through this invitation, many find a gentle presence that reassures them, time and time again, that they are guided, supported, and never truly alone.

Long ago, it was decided that every physical Earth human being would be accompanied by a main guide, known as the higher self, throughout their journey in physical form. This guide, often referred to as a Gatekeeper guardian, assists in guiding the ethereal human essence and soul plan energy into the physical Earth life and back to its source of creation. The higher self guide possesses extensive experience and deep understanding of life on Earth, gained through their own Earthly connections through a human experience.

In addition to the higher self, two additional celestial guides are present to provide support throughout the human's life. These celestial guides run errands for the higher self, offer support to the ethereal light energy body, and assist the team of celestial beings supporting the human individual. They source information, provide healing, and may offer guidance based on their own knowledge and experiences.

Throughout your life, other celestial guides may join the journey during significant life changes such as motherhood, fatherhood, education, health, and spiritual development. However, the three main celestial guides remain constant, offering guidance and support as needed. It is important to understand that these celestial guides are not here to control or make decisions for you. They are here to offer guidance and support, leaving the ultimate choices and decisions up to you as you control your own narrative.

The presence of our celestial star being friends, who serve as celestial guides, has significantly increased since World War Two. Their collaboration with humanity has been ongoing for a long time, with the goal of raising Earth's energies and contributing to the betterment of the universe. In recent times, more races of these beings have stepped forward to assist and monitor our Mother Earth. *(For more information, refer to my channelled book 'Spiritual Handbook'.)*

In recent years, various races of celestial beings have been communicating with us through different channels, such as trance communicators, light worker channellers, meditative states, and dream consciousness as well as Astral travel.

It is crucial to understand that these celestial beings are here to aid in our evolution and growth. They bring a wealth of knowledge and wisdom that can greatly benefit us. As we continue to elevate our consciousness and expand our awareness, we will be better prepared to receive their guidance and fully embrace their presence.

Who are your Celestial Guides?

Celestial beings are highly developed physical multi-dimensional transitional beings or light multi-transitional conscious beings. They are celestial beings not Aliens, as the term *"Alien"* is not recognised by them. They only use the word *"Alien"* when referring to species that work in darker energies of self-destruction, as this behaviour is alien to them. Your celestial guides wish to be known as celestial or universal guides, as they believe it is time for humans to understand them through new terminology.

A physical multi-dimensional transitional being that exists in the fifth and ninth dimensional high energies of the universe. They are telepathic and can transition mentally and physically into different forms to travel the universe and communicate telepathically with other beings. They can travel through energy streams, known as portals, to reach their desired destinations physically and telepathically as well as in star ships. Highly ascended physical beings live on a physical planet as a collective of beings in unity and light. Their science and technology are so advanced that it is beyond human understanding and is used to travel the universe.

The concept of a light ethereal conscious being is a fascinating one, as it exists in a multifaceted form existing in the tenth to twelfth dimensions. These beings possess the ability to create a physical presence that you can comprehend, as well as communicate telepathically and transition mentally and physically into various forms to travel the universe and interact with other celestial beings. They exist in different realms, dimensional energies, and collectives, making them truly unique and versatile.

A multi-dimensional transitional light conscious ethereal being can connect with a human form or other universal species as part of the universal connection program. Some beings choose to have only one human connection to better understand the human Earth form, while others are selected for multi-connections to bring light to Earth humans and aid in their ascension in the universe. They can also select to be a higher self guide to a physical form such as an Earth human.

It's important to trust that these celestial beings work collectively for their own learning and to enhance the vibration of humans and Earth. By understanding the existence of light and physical conscious celestial beings, you can expand your understanding of the universe and your place within it.

Here is a breakdown of the sort of celestial guides you have.

Inner guidance ring is a concept that has been around for centuries. It refers to the idea that each of you has a lifelong guide, known as your higher self, who oversees your journey from the moment of your ethereal self connection to your physical human form. This higher self is a silent guiding light that works in conjunction with a team of other celestial guides to aid you in your life's mission.

It's important to note that the Inner Guidance Ring is not a religious concept, but rather a spiritual one. It's about tapping into the wisdom and guidance that exists within you all and using it to navigate the challenges and opportunities that life presents. By cultivating a deeper connection with your inner guidance the soul plan, higher self and celestial guides, you can live more fulfilling and purposeful lives.

Unison celestial guides were first introduced as a crucial component of the new Earth Alliance following the Second World War. These celestial guides play a vital role in ensuring that all parties involved, including celestial guides, higher selves, soul plan base levels, and celestial guardians of Earth, work in harmony with one another and with their chosen humans.

The primary objective of unison celestial guides is to create a safe and conducive space where all parties can communicate effectively, regardless of their species or source of creation. This space of unison allows for seamless communication and collaboration, which is essential for achieving the desired outcomes.

Unison celestial guides are also responsible for overseeing the ethereal group connections of several humans, ensuring that they are aligned with their higher selves and soul plan energy. This ensures that humans are on the right path towards fulfilling their life's purpose and achieving their goals.

Earth human celestial guides – Please remember Earth humans are celestial beings as well. You can be guided by a physical Earth human who are essential to your spiritual journey. These humans embody deep spiritual wisdom and often can connect to the higher realms or dimensions. They may retain a strong connection to their divine quantum source essence, even in human form and the human will often feel different from an early age. They are deeply compassionate, intuitive, and aware of a greater purpose. These humans are not here for personal evolution, but to serve as bridges between the ethereal realms and earthly worlds, helping to raise consciousness and awaken love, healing, and unity across the planet.

Your human guide can take many forms, such as a leader of spiritual knowledge, holistic healer, nurturing grandmother, stranger, or a true friend who understands you on a deeper level. These human celestial guides have linked together with their ethereal light bodies and higher selves to help each other on their soul plan life journey. They are always communicating with each other and guiding their inner soul plan energy and human form.

Animal and Elemental celestial guides are additional celestial guides that you have in addition to your primary celestial guides. These ethereal celestial guides come from the animal and elemental kingdoms and provide grounding energy to assist you on your Earth journey. They present themselves as an animal for example a wolf or an elemental fairy reflecting the frequency needed for the human at the different stages of their life soul plan. They reside in a dimensional area known as *'Middle Earth'* while they work with you. Once their work with their Earth human is complete, they return to their dimensional existence and sources of creation. These elemental celestial guides can offer unique perspectives, insights and links you to Nature which is

Mother Earth's gift to us and can help you navigate life's challenges. By tapping into their wisdom, you can gain a deeper understanding of yourself and the world around you. You can also have physical form Earth animals like a pet dog whose life force and higher self is here to support your spiritual life journey.

Outer guidance ring - The outer guidance ring serves a variety of purposes. Some celestial guides are present to provide additional healing and assist in the pursuit of knowledge for the Earth life mission. Others are observers who are there to learn from the Earth life experience. These observers may eventually become one of your celestial guides or oversee another human as a guide. Although humans are often unaware of these celestial guides, they may be selected to communicate through trance or the channeller energy to impart their teachings to Earth. The outer guidance ring is a complex network of beings who are dedicated to supporting and guiding humanity on their journey. These celestial guides bring a wealth of knowledge and experience to the table, and their insights can be invaluable in helping you navigate the challenges of life.

Changing celestial guides - During your lifetime, it is common to have an average of six additional celestial guides at any given time. Some of these celestial guides may appear and disappear during different stages of your life. If you are a light worker, holistic healer or channeller, you may have a greater number of celestial guides to aid in your personal growth and life purpose. For those who have embraced this spiritual path, there are celestial guides eagerly waiting to join you on your journey towards spiritual awakening.

How our Celestial Guides Communicate with us - *Ten Levels of Channelling*

All communication from the celestial realms is through telepathic mind link, channelled communication. It can also involve the human sixth senses, (empathic third eye), smell, sight, hearing, touch, and taste. These energies can cause sensations in and around the human body that can change over time as you get used to them. Below is brief explanation on how each channelling energy system works.

1. Light worker channeller communication energy

Light worker channellers focus on bringing communication from the ethereal human essence that has passed over back to their source of creation.

They work in the clairvoyant energy with a higher more powerful energy vibration level. They have to keep themselves energised for a long period of time to keep their connection to source, the celestial realms. Their celestial guide team will help with this, harnessing the energy and using the energy around them to boost their connection. It takes dedication for the light worker channeller to achieve and sustain this level of energy that is needed.

The reason the higher energy is needed is because the essence of the loved ones that wish to communicate have not had the chance to blend with the light worker channeller energy before. It takes a lot of energy from the celestial realms to telepathically link and hold that communication process with the light worker channeller.

2. Psychic channeller energy links

All humans have a psychic energy level. This energy is considered by our celestial guides as high vibration, but not as high as needed for the clairvoyant connection. To be a psychic channeller you need to harness this connection energy, working alongside your celestial guide team. The working psychic channeller receives information about events and people from the ethereal vibration energy of a person, place, or object. A psychic can read a person's ethereal bodies energy picking up on health issues and may perceive past and present events, in that person's life. They should not be giving far off future life events as this is a false information as the human future can alter if needed for the greater good. If the recipient is given a potential future that is not truth to their life learning, it can steer them of their spiritual and soul plan path. The psychic reader can pick up on very near future guidance that helps the recipient of the message. All messages should be for the NOW to help the recipient to evaluate and move forward correctly on their life spiritual journey.

Psychic channellers will see the information in their mind's eye and feel energy and emotion to build their readings using all their senses. They are working more in the third dimension energy level, but also at times linking into guided information from a higher frequency of the fourth and fifth dimension energy. When this happens it is when the recipient's celestial guides, and the psychic channellers celestial guides communicate with each other to inspire the working psychic's mind. This ensures the correct information needed for the recipient is gathered and communicated. The psychic channeller will use the chosen tools like tarot or oracle cards or physical objects belonging to the recipient of the messages to inspire themselves with their celestial guides influencing their minds.

A clairvoyant light worker channeller when giving readings will drop into the psychic energy level if their energies are low. Some start readings off in the psychic energy slowly building up their energy and confidence to connect with the higher clairvoyant energies.

Each human has their own unique path of development along the light worker communication path. This is not to be criticised but understood by all that you are unique beings and develop your spiritual gift in different ways and pace.

3. Trance energy

The trance energy is a calmer more passive energy created by the celestial realms to allow inspiring words and communications from the celestial guides, human essences and observers of humanity. There are many different 'levels' and 'depths' of trance, between the states of *'Light Trance'* and *'Deep Trance'*. If you are drawn to trance you will develop to hold the trance energy for longer periods allowing longer conversations with the communicating celestial guides.

In **'Light Trance'** the sitter is often still aware of the room, they are in and what is going on around them. In the very lighter levels the sitter is inspired to speak with their eyes open, just connecting to the trance state. They can also do inspired inspiration writing which helps to strengthen the link with their celestial guides at this early stage. Their trance connection will get deeper as they progress on the trance journey. Some say it's like being in a meditative state of being.

'Deep Trance', is where a trance sitter can be nearly or completely totally unaware of anything that is happening with themselves and around them, they allow their conscious self to step aside, allowing the celestial communicator to communicate through their mind and voice. Some sitters will have some awareness but feel very distant from their normal reality. The truly deep trance state is often linked with the trance physical communication. *(If you seek further knowledge on Trance my book 'The Art of Trance' can provide this.)*

4. Channelling knowledge energy

Channelling knowledge energy is again a different calming energy that calmly builds strength over time. I am talking about a unique special energy that is created for the chosen celestial guides communicator(s) to build with their chosen human's energy field. This is the human knowledge facilitator predestined to channel written knowledge from the celestial beings to publish for humanities spiritual development and ascension while here on Earth.

A selected celestial guide will build with the selected human the channelling energy slowly. The reason it's done gradually is to build up the telepathic communication in the wakened state of being which one day will flow smoothly like a conversation between humans. If it is not done correctly the human mind cannot cope with a sudden build-up of energy and will reject the process. The celestial guide will start by inspiring their mind with words making the human feel they need to express them. The human will express in short bursts of time through written word or verbal recording in the early stages. They may also be guided to source information from their world net. As the human trusts its journey to channel from celestial beings, the celestial guide will build the energy up to a point when the telepathic conversation is free flowing and can be typed up as it comes in. Now because the human mind is not developed much beyond the 3D energy field of Earth this is often limited up to 30-minute bursts of channelling with rest in-between.

When a human reaches the fourth and fifth dimensional energy levels the celestial guide forgets about using the human minds knowledge and brings new knowledge to Earth not yet revealed to humanity. This takes TRUST from the human, if you doubt this remember all knowledge on Earth was once NEW from the quantum domains creative intelligence source.

To clear up any confusion, this channelling energy is different to the clairvoyant energy for giving messages. Light worker channellers get information for the recipient through short high energy bursts which can be a mixture of words in the head, visualisation and using the body sensory system. Through the development they learn to interpret them and with time it becomes a quicker smoother process. It is very rare for a light worker channeller to have free flowing conversation like an experienced channeller of knowledge would from their channelling celestial guides.

5. Meditation energy

Meditation energy is an energy designed for humanities physical make up and it heightens the senses. Over time you will notice subtle physical and mental changes in your human form when you meditate.

In meditation, you are shifting your awareness from the usual thought focus, of past and future to the now moment creating calmness in the mind. In daily activity, the mind is engaged in observing, discriminating, deciding, analysing, and accomplishing. Meditation gives you the opportunity to shift gears, let go of this focus and experience a more peaceful, silent state of being.

With practice many can reach such a calm state of mind they explain it like being in a void, often described as empty and black. This void state is wonderful for mental health and physical well-being. Our celestial guides do like to use this meditative state of being to give you downloads of ancient knowledge, light codes, healing energies and send you on a visualisation journey using your imagination energy to celestial places. Your celestial guides can often work with the chosen knowledge channellers we mentioned earlier in meditation to show them off world places, celestial truth in new knowledge and celestial beings.

If you feel the need to practice meditation it comes from an innate longing to see and think beyond the chaotic third dimensional world surrounding you. Meditation is used worldwide not just by the spiritual community. There are many types, and it is wise to take the time to find the right type of meditation and vibration for you.

6. Dream state energy

When a sleep, this dream state energy level allows our celestial guides to bring images and communication from loved ones in the celestial realms. It also allows them to bring the healing you need. Also channel knowledge and information to your subconscious mind. Have you heard of out of body experiences? The ethereal light body can go on journeys out of the human physical body for knowledge and new experiences in the universe. They will be guided by a celestial guide and other energy sources to what is needed for them. Many of you might not remember the healing experiences or downloads. But you will remember knowledge needed to share to humanity. This is also a great energy for the chosen human channeller for the guide to get information to them for their writing which is often in the visual form.

7. Healing energy

Healing energy comes in on a vibration of unconditional love from the *'Quantum Domain'* pure love energy source and with celestial beings that work in the light.

Energy healing goes back thousands of Earth years, the oldest form being under the umbrella of Shamanic healing. Shamanism is historically, often associated with Earth's indigenous and tribal societies and has persisted all over your world since its inception in ancient native cultures such as Siberian, Indian, Native American, South American and Aboriginals. It involves beliefs that shamans, with a connection to the other world and elementals, have the power to heal the sick, communicate with celestial beings, and escort souls of the dead to the afterlife. Some of the holistic healing practices of our world today have been developed from this ancient practice.

Some energy healing is hands-on healing where the holistic healer channels a wonderful high source of unconditional love energy. This can be with the hands physically placed on the human body or held in the ethereal human energy field. The celestial guides of both human parties work with the healer to send the healing through the recipient's body targeting the areas that need healing. In this process they send healing light energy in, while removing any unwanted darker energy out of the body. Our celestial guides have learnt through working with humans that different types of energy from various universal healing realms can help us.

8. Unison energy

Unison energy helps with communication in the universe between all celestial beings. It is an energy created to sustain an energy space where all celestial beings from all types of existence can meet and communicate with each other. It allows species from physical multi-dimensional transcendent to light conscious multi-dimensional transcendent beings to exist in the same space creating an energy to sustain them in their own energy of existence, like air. This is how your celestial guides can meet and create circles that help groups, workshops and individual light workers and leaders of spiritual knowledge. The space can be held in unison starship vehicles to a dimensional realm energy field. This will depend on the celestial guides home existences to what choice is made to base the unison energy meet space in.

9. Prayer energy

Prayer is a communication energy in the third dimension energy matrix connected to the human mind and their ethereal light body energy. It is a one-way telepathic communication wavelength like a radio signal.

All prayers are heard at celestial guide level through to the quantum domain source energy levels. The prayers will be answered if it will help the human's life journey or another human's journey. Communication from the quantum creative intelligence source will filter to the celestial guides, and they will help with any answer that needs to be given. This is a test for every human as it tests their religious faith if prayers are not answered.

When decisions are made to answer the prayer, the celestial guides will set the motion in place. They also will leave signs to comfort you they have heard you. The knowledge in my *'Magic of Spirit'* book will help you see their signs and understand the different facets of your spiritual journey.

10. Soul plan and higher self energy

I frequently remind myself that humans on Earth are celestial beings, also known as star people or star children. The difference between us and our celestial guides is we are vibrating at a lower frequency within the 3D energy spectrum, compared to celestial beings from the fifth to twelfth dimensions.

The higher self is either a light conscious being or a highly ascended physical being. They create a reflection of self for ethereal connection which we understand as the soul Plan. This energy communication connection is an internal mind to body communication. Your soul plan energy connects with a part of the brain near the pineal gland and crown chakra allowing communication energy transmitting to the higher self and vice a versa. While the soul is with the chosen human physical form it is the Sat-nav for the physical Earth journey. When a human being succeeds at this connection great things can occur for the spiritual journey. Have you heard of *'Soul Plan Connection'*? This is vital for the physical being incarnated into, to find its true self and purpose, and is a challenge in the Earth's third dimension energy. The challenge is for the human consciousness to have an open clarity of eternal awareness to connect to the soul base energy to trigger its life purpose. So, the human form must ascend out of the heavy third dimension energy towards the fifth dimension higher frequencies energy and make a mid-way connection for this to happen.

Many lessons will be learned from the individual's life's process of trying to achieve this. If you feel you have not connected to your soul plan, then this work is vital for you to undertake. This communication connection to the soul plan is your next transition but not many humans achieve this as they are spiritually unaware, and it is vital to the human ascension process. This is one of humanity's missing links.

An Explanation of the Ethereal Human Essence, Higher Self & Life Soul Plan

The **ethereal human essence** is a consciousness, a quantum, ethereal energy being that blends with the human foetus at the moment of conception on Earth. This life-giving force is born from the boundless love of the universal quantum domain, often referred to as the source of all creation or God energy. This intelligent ethereal light being's energy is intricately linked to the physical human form, connecting to everybody cell and the five senses and the sixth empathic sense. Together, these senses serve as powerful conduits of communication, connecting the conscious human mind to the essence of life itself.

This ethereal light essence can be newly formed or possess varying degrees of ascension, reflecting its ancient origins. Depending on their level of ascension within the quantum domains source collective, these ethereal celestial light beings are guided towards their next spiritual evolution. They have the choice to connect to a human on Earth, establishing a connection with a **higher self**, or to become the higher self guide, sharing a part of their essence for a new **soul plan**.

When a human passes away, the physical body returns to the Earth realms of one to three dimensions of energy, while the human essence ethereal light form undergoes healing in the Earth's energy layers, revealing its cosmic connection to its true ethereal light form and quantum source of creation. Once the ethereal human essence is freed from its earthly constraints and burdens, the ethereal essence of human life embarks on a journey back to the quantum source of the universe.

The ethereal light beings who have experienced life on Earth remain connected to Earth's energy, serving as celestial guides and messengers for loved ones known as light worker channellers. The love shared with others during their time on Earth is never lost, as the essence of humanity recognises and reunites with loved ones in the universal quantum domain through the pure frequency of love that once bound them together.

There has been some confusion surrounding the ethereal light body and its relationship to the higher self or soul plan. The ethereal light body is complex and can be connected to a physical form on Earth, as well as in other multi-dimensional time lines and various places in the universe simultaneously. The higher self is a multi-dimensional transitional physical or light being that takes on the responsibility of guiding a chosen human and overseeing all aspects of their existence, allowing the ethereal light body to fulfil its functions without impacting the physical human form it is linked to.

Prior to a human's conception, their higher self, ethereal light body, and celestial guides collaborate to devise a plan that will act as the guiding force behind the human individual's existence, the very essence of their existence that embodies who they truly are commonly known as a soul plan. The higher self assumes the role of the leader in crafting what our celestial guides describe as a reflection of self (soul plan), embedding this soul plan energy into the human physical body as an interconnected energy with human heart and brain.

All individuals on Earth possess a higher self and a soul plan, yet many go through life without recognising the energy of their soul plan and higher self. For those who believe in the existence of a soul plan, there is often a lack of understanding regarding this foundational energy. I aim to provide you with additional insight, as I believe you will experience enlightenment by tapping into this divine source of love energy. Connecting with this energy is crucial for any individual undergoing a *'Deep Core Healing'* process related to grief or for spiritual enlightenment.

The journey of the higher self soul plan energy involves various stages of transition as it embarks on its blending journey with the physical form it has chosen. This soul plan energy remains with you throughout your human life journey, serving as a guiding force along your life's path, akin to a GPS navigating you through life's twists and turns. This is what you would understand as your inner intuition.

Your higher self, which provided the soul plan energy, may be embarking on its first visit to a physical being as a guide, or it may have already been connected to multiple physical lives on different planets. As the Earth saying goes, they possess an *"Old Soul."* There are countless celestial beings in the universe participating in *"The Ethereal Connection Program"* or in human old terminology understanding the

"Incarnation Program", all seeking an experience with a human physical form. Through these experiences, they aim to learn and grow, bringing back new-found knowledge and experiences to their home worlds and points of collective existence. This accumulated wisdom is then added to the universal quantum knowledge library, serving as a valuable resource for those seeking further education and enlightenment.

When a soul plan energy connects with a chosen physical human form, it is referred to in our 3D understanding as incarnation in the old understanding of God's concept energy. This connection goes through various stages of transition, always linked to the higher self. While the origins of each soul plan connection may differ, the process of connection remains the same.

The original celestial form that creates the soul plan can range from a conscious ethereal light being to a highly ascended physical being, known as the soul plans higher self. This soul plan base reflects the energy of a being that has decided to guide a physical form on Earth to aid in the planet's ascension. This reflection of self is described as ethereal multi-dimensional transitional energy, which is essentially your soul plan life blue print.

During the moment of connection, the ordained transition to the chosen physical being's foetus occurs. The soul plan energy is a higher dimensional energy set in a special frequency that the young earthling in the womb can accept, establishing a connection to the Earth life. The Earth child exists in a heavier third-dimensional energy matrix, while the soul plan energy originates from a higher vibration energy form, such as the fifth-dimensional matrix or beyond. The slow blending process of vibration frequencies is crucial for the smooth transition of the soul plans energy, which can vary among individual universal species.

The day the young Earth being is born marks the soul plan energy second transition. As the baby takes its first breath, the soul plan energy base within strengthens into a higher frequency, initiating the journey of physical life alongside the ethereal body. Imagine your soul plan energy as a vessel suspended in a multi-dimensional energy field, behind your heart space gradually releasing itself to full strength.

As the human physical form evolves and matures on its life's journey, so does the strength of the soul plan energy. The soul plan energy possesses the wisdom necessary for the young being's journey, originating from a higher source. Picture a silver energy thread serving as a direct line, always connected to the soul plan so it can reach its true source of guidance. This silver energy thread also serves as a conduit for the higher self to observe its soul plan reflection within the human form.

At a certain point in each human being's life journey, a harmonisation of soul plan frequencies and physical body takes place. This moment varies for each Earth being and species - have you ever heard a sixty-year-old human say, *"But I feel like I'm thirty-two inside"*? This sensation of inner age reflects the soul plans true maturing age when it fully balanced within the human, which remains constant until a final third transition stage occurs. This stage varies for each physical being chosen for the connection process, depending on their life mission. **How old do you feel inside?**

As the human form nears the end of its life, the soul plan energy, begins to prepare for the transition back to the higher self, marking the third stage of this transformative process. During this time, the higher self and celestial guides patiently await the release of the soul plans energy along with the ethereal human essence, from physical human form and the earthly realm.

Once this transition occurs, the soul plan energy which is full of knowledge, is aided by the ethereal human essence, higher self and celestial guides, journeys back to its higher self. This moment signifies the near completion of the final transition. Depending on the experiences outlined in the higher self's soul plan and the ethereal human essence's journey on Earth, healing may be necessary before fully departing from the earthly realm.

The final completion phase occurs when all aspects are healed, rebalanced, and returned to their original quantum source in the universe, signifying a harmonious reunion within the cosmos.

I hope this explanation sheds light on your true essence and the intricate transition processes of the soul plan energy, higher self and ethereal human essence. By establishing a genuine connection with your soul plan energy, you can navigate through life with ease, discovering your true path and authentic self.

I know living in alignment with the light ethereal body, higher self, and soul plan is not about avoiding the human experience but about navigating it with mindfulness. It involves recognising the sacredness of life, listening to your intuition, and making choices based on love rather than fear. Every moment, even the difficult ones, is a piece of a larger picture that we are a part of.

We are not defined solely by our physical bodies or the challenges we face. Our existence extends beyond this current lifetime. It is through embracing our human experiences, including our bodies, emotions, and struggles, that we come to realise our true divine essence.

Chapter three

Insight into Deep Core Healing

Human Perspective

I bring you this guidance to share how our celestial guides view humanity from a higher-dimensional perspective. Humanity lives within a three-dimensional matrix of vibration, an energy far heavier than the higher-frequency realms celestial guides channel from. Mother Earth, too, holds many layers of dimensional vibration, yet she currently pulses in a 3D frequency overlapped by higher energetic layers. She is weighed down by the fear energy humanity generates, and this dense vibration shapes a slow, heavy reality that many struggle to move through. It creates a fear-based existence in which people long for change but feel as if they are climbing an endless hill. This leads to disillusionment, self-doubt, anxiety, and fear of both the past and the future. Heavy 3D energy forms a barrier that blocks lighter, higher-frequency love energy, the vibration frequency that dissolves fear.

Right now, I am working with celestial beings to help humanity shift out of this dense 3D frequency. A crucial part of this change begins with how you see yourself and your world. Your perspective shapes your life story and how you wish to be seen. As you grow up and begin making your own decisions, you form a persona shaped by external influences, beliefs, and emotional experiences. Your body is energy, your thoughts are energy, your ethereal auric field is energy, and together they form your unique vibrational signature within the 3D matrix.

For centuries, ethereally connected celestial light bodies that connected with the physical human form at birth on Earth primarily were here to learn for self within these heavy energies. But after the last world war, everything changed. Humanity was moving toward self-destruction, and the overseers of Earth called upon celestial beings from across the universe to intervene. Many of them came as observers, celestial guides, and choose to ethereally connect to a human physical form. They shifted from simply gathering lessons for their own ascension to actively supporting humanity's survival and growth.

From this work, they identified what humanity must now remember:

• You are connected to *The Quantum Source* from birth.
• You must rediscover the soul plan, the higher self, and intuition.
• You must uncover your true self and your Earth missions.
• You must understand dimensional existence and the energetic realms beyond physical 3D reality.
• You must learn about the shift into 5D multi-dimensional consciousness.
• You must reconnect with ancient Earth wisdom returning at this time to help humanity heal.
• You must understand the alliances between ascension beings and Earth.
• You must understand the 2019 awakening and why it occurred.

- You must learn to live without fear and self-doubt.
- Above all, you must change your perspective.

Your own next stage of ascension begins when you take responsibility for your life, question your beliefs, and release false perspectives.

Here is something else to consider. Scientists and astrologers see the universe from a strictly 3D viewpoint. When a telescope observes a distant galaxy, the interpretation is limited by a 3D understanding. They cannot see the dimensional layers, the energy grids, the harmonic tones, or the realms of life that exist beyond 3D physical form.

A recent experience illustrates this. I met a professor who studies how viruses affect the human body. When I asked him about celestial beings, life after death, self-healing, and the higher self and soul plan, he replied that he would not believe anything without proof. I shared some of my experiences but quickly realised he needed his own direct experience to believe. This is common in the 3D reality.

I explained to him how limited the human mind becomes when confined to 3D thinking. I encouraged him, with all his intelligence, to think beyond what he can physically see. He stared at me in silence, as though I were otherworldly. Later I realised this moment was exactly what my celestial guides had been teaching me; intelligence alone does not free the mind from 3D limitations. Yet I know the **human mind *can* expand**. Great thinkers like Stephen Hawking demonstrated the ability to step outside restrictive thought patterns, proving there is hope for humanity.

When I asked my celestial guides how humanity can truly change, their answer was simple: *"Children must be raised with mindfulness, meditation, self-healing, and sound healing woven into their education. Earth babies are born open and connected to higher quantum intelligence. If they grow up with spiritual awareness alongside their 3D schooling, their minds will expand naturally. Those with high intelligence and higher spiritual understanding will evolve further, establishing communication with celestial species and accessing universal knowledge.*

You are a telepathic race, capable of hearing higher guidance. Many already do. But without spiritual understanding, this ability is often misunderstood. Light workers with ascended minds, those who vibrate in 4D to 6D frequencies, recognise and trust this communication."

It makes you think, does it not?

Human life V's Spiritual Development

Below are two truth lifelines of two humans showing how they live the planned human life events designed to trigger the spiritual awakening of that individual.

This is a brief description of two humans' life's showing their human life alongside the spiritual ascension development. They highlight where they have had key healing experiences with the three-dimensional human clinic medicine and holistic healing. The examples are also to show you how the perspective of your life's can be altered through other human and Earth experiences.

Human example A
Female
Born 1960
Here celestial guides tells her story.

- Mother was unmarried and father unknown - human A placed for adoption at six weeks old.
- Adopted into a family that had struggled to have children of their own. She had two brothers by her adoptive parents, and she was the middle child.
- Early childhood was safe and strict. Spiritually she did not enjoy Sunday school and felt out of place from an early age. She was told she was adopted but did not have much understanding of it in the early stages of childhood. She had a feeling of being out of place, which was a mixture of her adoption and her ability to stay tuned to higher energies, but she had no understanding at that age as there was no human guidance to help her. She was bullied and teased at school for her red hair colour, freckles and that her father taught at her school.
- From the age of thirteen she experienced her first connection with the ethereal humans' essences passed over, this happened when on holiday in an old cottage. The energy of a murdered woman was recorded in the energy of the building; she was fearful at the time of this new phenomenon in her life. Also, she struggled with her relationship with her adoptive mother who was a very indoctrinating person and mentally dominated her.
- From aged fourteen to nineteen she was aware of UFO's and celestial beings and was drawn to knowledge on this subject.

She also experienced a vision back in time of a previous life and physical contact with a ethereal presence in a pub. She was also experiencing a dream that took her back in time, and she felt she had been there and lived that life. *(This dream was a connection to a past life that was a planned trigger point for her spiritual journey)*. Her parents had become drinkers, and she tried to deal with this in daily life. Depression and an attempt of taking her own life also featured in this time period. She was sexually molested at fourteen by a neighbor. At the age of nineteen she met her life partner and universal ethereal companion. Her parents did not approve of her partner which caused friction. She left home to be with him and became estranged from her parents over the years. Depression reared its head again and she sought medical advice and was placed on drugs for it for a few months. The happiness and safety she found with her partner helped to heal her to a certain point. And move on with her life.

- From age twenty to thirty-two. she completed collage and her life took her to Cheltenham. She got a good job in a marketing company but suffered four years of bullying in the workplace. She married at the age of twenty-five. The relationship with her parents stayed strained even on her wedding day. She distanced herself from her parents to protect herself from the pain the strained relationship had on her. Not a form of healing but self-preservation we see a lot of humans do. Her life and work took her to Bradford and Edinburgh. In her late twenties she had an early miscarriage, which was an unplanned baby. The energy of this light being that briefly connected with the Earth plane will be with her through her life spiritually. At the age of thirty-two she had the calling to have a child, she had some experiences of seeing and sensing spirit which kept her interest in the subject.

- Age thirty-three to forty-five. At the age of thirty-three she gave birth to a son in Edinburgh. She suffered mild postnatal depression and felt isolated. Her husband moved jobs to the Midlands where their families lived. This was a planned preordained move as they would be needed by family at this time. At the age of thirty-six and a half she gives birth to a second son, and she struggled with her mental health after he was born. Her husband's brother emigrated to Canada and his sister to America. Her father in-law passed away, and her adoptive father was very ill but pulled through. Meanwhile she was training online to be a garden designer. On top of this her husband's mother developed a blood cancer disorder. At the age of 38 she moved to Bristol UK through her husband's job, and she had a break down that led to suicidal thoughts. She was diagnosed with severe postnatal depression. A lot of factors led to this, but her main thoughts through counseling, was her depression was related to her childhood and early adult hood and her relationship with her adopted mother. A medical professional told her she had been mentally abused by her mother and the deep-set memories of this had affected her after her second child. She then moved forward in this reality belief system which narrowed her perspective to other life options and new possibility's. Her predicted pre-life timeline estimated two to three years for full recovery from this period of depression, but it took four and a half years. It was planned at the end of this postnatal depression her spiritual path would be triggered. During the four and a half years of healing through human clinical treatment and drugs, she finished training as garden designer and worked part time in this role. She was also a school governor and became a chair of governors, using her energies to give to others. As to her spiritual path she read about angels and was still fascinated by UFOs.

- Age forty-six to sixty-two. In her early forty's she was diagnosed with a condition called Fibromyalgia. A condition that in the future was to show her how your body develops illnesses when holding onto dark memories and the deep core energies residues. When she was forty-seven her husband set up a home marketing business and in 2007, they move it out the family home to an office space in 2008. This led to a friendship with a light worker channeller who had a healing business next to theirs. She struck up a friendship and told her about her spiritual experiences, UFOs, and her repetitive dream of another life. Her light worker friend suggested a past life regression. She was not keen and to be honest she was afraid about a past life regression, but over a few months and our guidance she had one.

- This was the window of opportunity we had been waiting for. She stepped through her first spiritual open door into the spiritual connection on her path to spiritual ascension on Earth. Her celestial guide team, then could guide her to receive more healing to move forward with us on this spiritual connection path. This led her to doing Reiki one and two when she was fifty-one and she sat in a Reiki and meditation circle for a couple of years. This was a time where she had to face her feeing's about her adoptive mother and her birth mother. A lot of self-healing and acceptance was granted, enough to allow her to work with us in the Light. She still held heavier energies around the memories, but healing helps to shift this to appoint you can consciously function in acceptance and connect to the divine source of healing to give to others. This time period also led to an introduction to light worker communication. Over a couple of years, she traveled the path of developing her light worker channeling communication skills which led to an introduction to trance. The trance journey led to her celestial guides to triggering a channeling connection so she could fulfill her path of writing books channeled by us. She also developed a holistic business which became her full-time job in her late fifties.

During this busy spiritual time of development, she of course was living her human life. Bringing up two sons and coping with her husband who had gone partially sighted. She conquered Fibromyalgia, came of her drugs and self-healed through mind over body and meditation. After her adoptive father died, she decided to seek out her birth family. She had to cope with rejection from her birth mother again. But she did find comfort in getting to know her uncle and one of her cousins. We sent her birth grandmothers human essence energy to her through a light worker communicator to let her know she would never see her birth mother in this Earth lifetime. This was so her human side could except this and heal so lighten her energies.

By 2016 her sons had left home and for financial security they moved to South Wales so they could become mortgage free. This was a preplanned destiny and helped to shift her energies into a safe space with less worry. She re-established her business and carried on working with us channeling books. It is in the early days of living in South Wales, UK, her celestial guide team bought her a new guide called John. He is a highly ascended light being from the Salcaritons - bringing her amazing communication and teachings to share with others. Her celestial guides realised as did her higher self soul plan base that they needed to bring the next stage of her healing, **Deep Core Healing**. This led them to guiding her to write about herself through her diary's she kept from the age of thirteen to twenty. This explored the false perspective belief system she had lived in for forty years of her life. The book allowed for her to face the truth and heal and release the **negative deep core energy in her cells** and energy field left from earlier healing. She then had a spiritual rest for a few weeks and human holiday allowing herself to adjust. This Deep Core Healing released her conscious mind and body into the next stage of spiritual journey on Earth. It now means she is very highly attuned to the celestial beings that communicate and guide her. The Deep Core Healing allowed her to revisit her childhood and reanalyse these past events. She was shocked to realise she had thrived for forty years on the energy of wanting to be the victim of mental abuse to be true. Blaming her adoptive mother for her bad mental health and always being the victim. Through her analysing her youth through her dairies she came to a new positive conclusion that shifted the dark emerging creating

Deep Core Healing. She is now on a higher vibration for her human health and spiritual work. ***She had changed her perspective***.

To conclude this section of her life the Deep Core Healing will allow us to bring further new knowledge to Earth through channeling her our words.

Human example B
Female
Born 1982

- Born into a family of a mum, dad and at the time of birth, an older brother of three and half years chosen on her soul plan contract for spiritual growth.
- Early childhood was a mixture of happy and not so happy memories. She had some problems with school where a teacher was bullying her for not being able to hold information in and her mum had to step in. Even though she had friends around her, she felt very much isolated much of the time. She could sense ethereal light energies in her home that would scare her at a young age as she never knew or understood from an early age what it was that she was sensing at the bottom of her home stairs. She was a sensitive person and sometimes her mum spoke for her instead of allowing her the space to speak for herself as she was so shy. She recalls many pleasant memories around her uncle's home in north Wales, especially sitting in the big window and glancing out over the sea. Both parents worked full time, and she spent a lot of time in the care of other families whose mothers were not the nicest of people.

- From the age of thirteen she still struggled to fit in at school and didn't really want to be there. She struggled learning the way the schools taught and didn't want to know. Many times, she wrote about aliens in her school stories and was told she had an amazing imagination. The alien influence perhaps came from her dad who was fascinated with the subject. Little did she know back then her celestial guides influenced her mind on the UFO subject as she had come here to seek this knowledge as part of her ascension.
- From the age fourteen to nineteen she was starting to find her own personality and noticing that her dad's temper could go from 0-60 and sometimes hid upstairs out the way of the shouting. Her brother was also bullying her badly and her dad would pin him up against the door some days as he didn't know when to stop. She wasn't allowed to go out with her friends as much as she'd like as her parents didn't have much money. Or they would say no, or she would have to come in a lot earlier than the other children, even at the age of 16. As she grew older, she realised that she could do some training and get a practical job from her electronics skills learnt in a factory.
- From the age of twenty to thirty-two she started to venture out more with her friends and was becoming more social and spending less time on the computer playing games. Around the age of 24 she had a relationship with a man who was extremely manipulative due to having a mother who was an alcoholic which caused him mental health problems that were projected onto others. She and her family went through an ordeal with her partner which left her with

mental and physical scarring. With no healing she moved on with her life burying all her emotions.

- She eventually moved on into a new job working in a biscuit factory where she made new friends on top of her old friends. She had a relationship with one of her younger childhood friends around the age of 29 who would treat her like trash when it suited him which lasted for a year. At the age of thirty-one, she met someone new who appeared to be charming in the beginning. She had gotten a feeling that she had felt before in a past toxic relationship, yet she ignored it, her soul plan based intuition. At this point she was still living at home with her parents and became pregnant with her daughter which was a huge surprise but a feeling that this was part of her life's path.

- Around the second year after her daughter being born, she was beginning to become curious about tarot cards. She was invited to a small development circle by a medium who suggested she had physic skills. She was also studying when her daughter was at a young age as she wanted to prove to herself that she could pass her English GCSE, and this is when she learned that she was dyslexic.

Her daughter's dad came back in on the scene for a while after she worried about not having a dad figure in her daughter's life. She had to chase him through the child maintenance system as he had vanished off the scene and denied being her daughters' father.

From age thirty-three to present. As she began to start to get her life back on track, she was studying counselling, through this she started to discover who she really was. This was the start of Deep Core Healing process. One day she was drawn to a lady who gave her a reading at a spiritual fair. She joined in on some of her spiritual development workshops and enjoyed them greatly and for the first time, felt like she belonged somewhere. This was a big phase of her spiritual journey and as she had been through a healing phase from her human life through her counselling journey, she had cleared negative energy allowing us to step into guide her.

Much of her memories around the time of the events that unfolded around her daughter, her dad and herself and what happened altogether, are fragmented. This caused a confused perspective on her reality. This is because the human mind cannot process a huge amount in one go, so the mind shuts down and fragments the memories. You then live in a false perspective of your reality, and this is when Deep Core Healing will clear this deep negative energy.

Around the age of thirty-four to thirty-five the mental abuse towards her from her daughter's father and trying to help another family member deal with a psychopath had mentally and physically exhausted her, in the end, she had an emotional break down. This was the start of consciously becoming aware of number signs appearing and later learning that the numbers would help her to connect with her celestial guides and she started to build herself back up slowly with help from friends, family, and professional clinical help. She went through an ordeal of trying many different anti-depressant meds that had horrendous side effects until finding the right one. This is an example of human clinical medicine working alongside the start of spiritual enlightenment.

As she gradually started to get herself back up on her feet, she decided to study psychology in the form of NLP (Neuro-Linguistic Programming). For the first time in a while, it was something positive that she had chosen to do for herself to better her future for herself and daughter.

She studied many courses in the one year around 2019 including computers at the beginning of the year. Business Wales courses, three more NLP courses without having holidays in between and ended up burning out for 3 months. But her recovery was quicker this time around due to having time line therapy on the coaching course. She experienced a moment with the tutor who gaslighted her and denied what she had said the day before only to realise later that they had both been triggered as they were both mirroring passed versions to each other known as transitional analysis in psychology but spiritually known as a soul growth exchange.

In 2019 she also felt a knowing that something was going to happen, not quite sure when and started to put small amounts of food away on her weekly shopping and even started to warn people and felt crazy for doing so. She spoke to her spiritual mentor who was doing the same and so made her feel a little more at ease. She also started to do things like taking her daughter to London and pushed past her comfort zones and was so proud of doing so. She was given money off one of her parents and got a tattoo to remind her of how far she had come and that she could get through anything that came in.

Her celestial guides were now communicating more through the numbers and as she went into the spiritual awakening that came in December 2019, she came off her anti-depressants whilst being away from work and the pace of life had slowed down. She felt a lot of pressure emotionally as she knew she had to take good care of herself and her daughter as best she could through the experience but was grateful, she had her celestial guides along the way supporting her.

She was also extremely lucky that she visited many places during these two years, including going back to the cottage she once went on holiday as a child, she went with her brother who could recall more memories of this past visit than she did.

Rolling onto to the present time where she is now in her early forties and has learned A LOT around herself and others. She is re-learning healthy boundaries not only with herself and others but also with her spirit team as she has quite a few groups now who love to help her.

She had a relapse early 2022 due to many reasons, complex trauma, PTSD and losing her own identity after being caught up in things that had a negative influence at the same time of realizing a lot of truths. She also felt isolated and overwhelmed as she felt that same feeling in April 2022 as she once felt in August 2019. This time it was more conscious awareness around a war that was announced but at the same time, knowing that humanity was in the transition period of the great awakening that so many had prophesized. She also went back onto anti-depressants and noticed this time around that the side effects made things worse and that doing mindset working with her friend who was a coach, working with her celestial guides and her spiritual mentor had much more of a positive effect along with walking in nature. This relapse was a process she had to go through as the healing recovery was quicker, and it showed her how far she had come on her life's journey.

She fell into a new relationship and knew from the beginning it felt wrong and for a while carried on out of the fear of being alone once more and isolated. She listened to her gut feeling that she had felt in two previous relationships and had ignored it, but this time she wasn't going to. She now had a duty of care for her daughter and soon realised that as she let go of this person, the people she was now drawing into her life had more respect and love and compassion for her.

Deep down, she knew that he was a life lesson for soul plan growth. She is also starting to build back up and is quite stubborn when it comes to slowing down. She has learnt to deal with issues that are around so many patterns that show up in her life and doing the best she can with what she has. Even though she is going through Deep Core Healing, she knows deep down that with time, all will work out for the best if she just keeps putting one foot in front of the other and trusting her life's path. She is grateful for all the life lessons that have been presented as she wouldn't be where she is today and starting up a coaching business to help others.

She is also grateful that her mentor and mentors' celestial guides helped her to push through barriers to get her book out into the world after a battle with herself and baring her soul to those who would read it. What she did not realise was **this book was part of her Deep Core Healing process**. Scared of moving forward as she was experiencing so much pain at the same time but was lucky that her mentor and her celestial guides kept her accountable and to get the book out into the public domain. This was a key time on human B's ascension path and shows how Deep Core Healing can work, triggering the human to face up to the past so they can heal and move forward on their Earth ascension path.

She still has her struggles and battles each day, good and bad days, sometimes questioning why life has been so tough and what on earth she had agreed to on her soul plan contract before coming here.

Her celestial guides asked her to write a second book of her human life, spiritual growth and Deep Core Healing, so far on Earth. She has found this has been a challenge for her and wants nothing more than peace of mind and body and to build a bright future for herself and daughter. This phase of healing for her through her book will open new powerful cosmic doors for her spiritual growth and experiences here on your Earth. Also enhancing her connection with the quantum source and future channeling.

As you read these two human examples of human life with spiritual life balance you might recognise yourself in the words. Remember every human life is unique and different. But many of the spiritual teachings and chosen life lessons can be recognised by many but will be different in various stages of your life.

A combination of therapies was used to help **Human B** on her healing ascension path. These were Reflexology, Reiki, NLP, Hypnosis, Trance, Time line Therapy and having a spiritual mentor to talk to. I will cover some of these in for you to understand and relate to. With her various treatments her mind and body healed opening the way to truth and a new perspective on her life.

Every step listed below takes hard work and commitment from you to achieve as you have to change a lifetime of old habits. Once you take the decision to change your perspective, we can help you on this journey. Every human that starts a spiritual journey of learning will have a new guide working with their other celestial guides to help them ascend on the Earth life.

Step 1: Look at your thought patterns: are you living in the old structure reality of existence in a world of hate, depression, sickness, fear, and negativity? Do you find when you find what you think is love you destroy it? Are you on a self-destruct reality path? Yes! Trust small steps of reviewing your life and how you can change for the better will make the difference. Place reminders in your home, work, car and in fact everywhere you go that positive thoughts bring love into your life.

Step 2: Learn to love yourself as you are, knowing positive changes will help you grow to be a better person. Set yourself daily affirmations of how wonderful you are repeat this daily.

Step 3: Learn meditation and mindfulness. This will still your mind and bring you clarity and better health through relaxation.

Step 4: Learn to evaluate yourself weekly. Do not be hard on yourself just set small goals of how you can improve your life for the better. For example, look at your food and drink intake and how much you exercise. What person do you want to be this time next year? How will you achieve this? Imagine you are in the new positive reality you want to achieve for yourself.

Step 5: Trust the spiritual journey. You have celestial guides that wish to help you change and achieve your spiritual life mission of positive change while here on Earth. Talk to them and ask them for help.

Step 6: Seek a spiritual Earth human mentor to guide you through this journey

Step 7: As you achieve your goals of change for the better, YOU must pat yourself on the back at your positive progress. Then take a leap of faith and stride forward in life to your new positive loving reality future.

This mission of perspective alteration will change humanity; humans will start to shift their own unique vibrational energy footprint to the lighter fourth and fifth dimensional energies. This will open up doors of universal knowledge as your new higher frequency perspective will see the true cosmic reality. Then BOOM humanity on Earth will then unite with the many ascension celestial species through the universe that have an alliance with Earth through the overseers. Humanity will live among the many star systems and help many other species to ascend.

Your celestial guides hope you except this mission of changing your perspective as they are fully committed to this mission if you choose to except it. They ask when excepted you teach this new perspective to the children of your world.

Life can be the fairy tale you wish to make it. You deserve happiness and success, and this can all be achieved while existing in a kind loving positive energy of existence.

Be the change.

Be the positive ending.

Be the inspirer for others to follow.

Chapter four

The Human Body is a Self-healing Machine

Ancient Codes

Your physical body is a remarkable regenerative machine encoded with ancient healing wisdom. Explore grounding, empathy, and emotional energetic links that influence well-being on body, mind, and soul plan levels.

Your physical body is far more than a biological organism operating through chemistry and cellular intelligence. It is a multi-dimensional vessel, encoded with ancient cosmic knowledge and designed to regenerate, rebalance, and heal itself on physical, emotional, mental, and spiritual levels. To walk the Deep Core Healing path is to remember that healing begins not outside of you, but from the inner hologram of who you truly are a quantum energetic being with limitless potential.

In this chapter we explore the ancient DNA codes, the empathic consciousness of the human body, and foundational practices such as grounding and energetic regulation. These teachings reconnect you with the living intelligence present within your cells, your sixth sense, and your link to Mother Earth herself.

The Ancient Codes within the Human Body

The human body is a delicately designed framework of cells, energy, and memory. Modern science understands DNA primarily as a biological instruction system determining physical traits and personality tendencies, but much more remains unseen.

Within your DNA lies ancient cosmic coding, written long before the human species entered its current density of reality. These codes contain spiritual memory, healing intelligence, and knowledge from eras when humanity existed in a higher dimensional state, functioning through a twelve-strand DNA system instead of two.

This multi-dimensional DNA cannot yet be measured by current scientific tools, but it can be felt, activated, and remembered through the empathic sensory system, the sixth sense.

Many are awakening now because humanity has entered a profound ascension cycle the *Quantum Era*. These ancient codes are stirring, unlocking dormant abilities, deeper intuition, and a heightened sense of purpose. Every human being alive today is here to contribute to planetary evolution, whether consciously aware or gradually awakening to it.

Your mission is not only personal healing, but also planetary.

You are here to help:

• Restore compassion

• Remember unity

• Embody higher consciousness

• Teach the generations who follow

Long ago Earth existed in a high-vibrational 5D state, filled with harmony and purity. Over time, as conscious beings incarnated and collective fear, ego, and separation consciousness deepened, Mother Earth shifted into a heavier 3D vibration. This shift created an imbalance, one that humanity now has the power to correct.

Mother Earth cries out for healing, not in punishment, but in invitation. The solution is not abandonment of the planet but a conscious return to unity consciousness, responsibility, and love. Each human who raises their vibration contributes to the strengthening of the whole.

Your body, being part of Mother Earth, responds to this transformation. Every cell is fuelled not only by food and water, but by:

- Light

- Colour

- Unconditional love

- Harmonic vibration

- Spiritual intention

Healing begins when you recognise yourself as energy.

The Empathic Link - The Sixth Sense Remembered

Every human is born empathic. Empathy is not a personality trait, it is a spiritual sensory system, enabling you to attune to the emotional, energetic, and vibrational quantum fields around you.

Your five senses, sight, sound, touch, taste, and smell, are governed by your physical interface. Your sixth sense, often depicted in ancient symbolic art as the "Third Eye," is governed by your higher consciousness and soul plan connection.

This empathic energy allows you to sense:

• Other peoples' emotional states

• The vibrational energy of places

• Unspoken truths

• The presence of higher celestial beings

• Subtle energetic changes in yourself and others

Signs of an active empathic system include:

• Absorbing others' emotions

• Deep compassion

• Sensing hidden pain or truth

• Strangers confiding in you

• Connection to animals and children

• Vivid dreams and inter-dimensional memories

• Emotional overwhelm in crowded spaces

• A desire to help or heal

Many human empaths shut down their gift early in life because the 3D world does not yet teach energetic boundaries. Without training, the ethereal empathic body absorbs emotional and energetic debris from others, leading to:

• Anxiety

• Fatigue

• Depression

• Self-doubt

• Confusion

• Feeling *"different"* or isolated

• Not belonging

Deep Core Healing re-activates the empathic system in a protected, stabilised way. As your vibration rises, you become able to decode what you sense without absorbing it, allowing you to work as a healer, intuitive, guide with balance and clarity.

This is why connection to celestial guides is essential, they help regulate the empathic system and clear the emotional residue collected from others.

Light Workers and Empaths in Service

Light workers on Earth are humans who have a soul plan destination to assist humanity's evolution. They feel a deep inner calling to uplift others, awaken consciousness, and support healing on both personal and planetary levels.

A Light worker or empath can sense when another human is in emotional, physical, or energetic distress. Guided by higher intuition and supported by their celestial guide spiritual team, they naturally step into a vibration of compassion. Through this elevated state, they are able to:

• Intuitively recognise the needs of others

• Remain centred without becoming overwhelmed by emotional pain

• Serve as a stabilising presence in turbulent moments

• Channel healing energy and higher light frequencies where needed

• Communicate to off world celestial beings

Light workers appear in many forms: trance communicators, energy healers, channellers, holistic practitioners, therapists, teachers, mentors, medical carers and everyday humans who carry a profoundly compassionate nature.

However, sensitivity is both a gift and a responsibility. Without proper grounding, emotional regulation, and regular energetic clearing, the ethereal empathic system can become overloaded. When this happens, the body and mind begin to strain under the weight of absorbed emotions and unprocessed energy.

A Light worker's service becomes sustainable only when they:

• Honour their own healing as much as others

• Remain grounded in the physical body

• Clear emotional and energetic residue regularly

• Maintain strong boundaries

• Listen to their higher guidance and intuition

When these foundations are in place, the Light worker becomes a powerful channel of compassion, stability, and ascension light on Earth, not by force, but simply by being aligned with their true cosmic quantum nature.

Grounding - Returning to Mother Earth

In a human high-frequency body, grounding is not optional, it is vital. Grounding rebalances your nervous system, returns scattered energy to Mother Earth, and strengthens your physical, ethereal and emotional stability. Modern lifestyles disconnect humans from Mother Earth. Plastic-soled shoes, constant technology exposure, and indoor living prevent the body from exchanging charge with the planet. Historically, leather shoes and bare feet allowed this exchange, maintaining energetic flow.

Un-grounded individuals often experience:

• Mental fog

• Emotional instability

• Feeling *"distant"* or *"disconnected"*

• Weakened energy systems

• Difficulty manifesting or staying focused

When you embark on a Deep Core Healing journey your energies will fluctuate as the heavier energy disperses it will be replaced with higher frequency light energy, so grounding often will help your healing journey. Grounding restores clarity, peace, and stability.

There is a grounding mediation in Chapter six.

Chapter five

Healing Choices for Humanity

Human Clinical Medical Treatment

In ancient times of humanity holistic healing through energy healing and natural herbs was used to heal the human body and mind.

Over the last one hundred and fifty years the medical professionals of Earth have advanced creating lifesaving surgery, cancer cures and human made drugs such as antibiotics.

Medical treatment is the attempted remediation of a health problem, usually following a medical diagnosis. When I talk about medical treatment, I am talking from the human cold to more serious diseases, illnesses like cancer and surgical operations. This will include the man-made drugs to kill germs and relieve pain.

You can probably preempt what I am going to say. If humanity had developed a higher spiritual understanding instead of fear leading to war, self-destruction, and persecution off others, our health and healing practices would mainly be holistic in our modern day. But this is how your future can be trusting my words to help you change your restricted mindset. To achieve Deep Core Healing at this time in our three-dimensional matrix society, with the humans not yet existing in the lighter higher vibration, it will be a blend of our modern clinical medicine and holistic therapy. For those humans further along the spiritual journey they will start to shed the need for our modern medicine as they will be healing at a higher frequency level of existence. We now lead on to a brief explanation of your holistic choices.

Holistic Healing Choices

Holistic therapy addresses the mind, body, and ethereal light self to support health and healing. They are often known to you as alternative therapies or holistic medicine. They are a mixture of nature's herbal medicine, energy hands on healing, massage, sound energy healing and spiritual counselling. Holistic healing focuses on the person as a whole and the mind sets how the body feels, which in turn effects the ethereal light body energy. I will lay out some holistic healing methods for you and how they can help you. Having this knowledge will help you understand how holistic healing can help you heal. When you make the choice to heal yourself and set that intention to do so, your celestial guides will guide you to the appropriate ones that will benefit you the most at that time on your life's journey.

Human holistic treatment can also include diet and exercise advice, psychotherapy, relationship, and spiritual counseling. These can run long aside complementary and alternative therapies.

For example, types of **complementary therapies** can be Acupuncture, Yoga, Tai chi and Qigong, Meditation, Music and art therapy, Massage, Physical activity, and Nutrition.

Examples of **Alternative therapies** are Acupuncture, Alternative medical systems like Traditional Chinese Medicine, Aromatherapy, Herbal remedies, Homeopathy and Hypnotherapy.

If you have picked up this book to look at alternative healing methods and are on the human medical drugs, it is sensible to speak to your doctor. Our celestial guides recognise in the 3D reality the modern medicine is how humanity sees it can heal itself, but the two can work alongside each other. As you travel the holistic healing journey the human modern medical needs will fade, and you will exist without the human made clinical drugs as you heal your body and mind.

All holistic healing should be done in a safe quiet space for your comfort allowing a wonderful experience for the healer and the recipient.

Energy Healing

I will start with energy healing. This goes back thousands of Earth years, the oldest form being under the umbrella of Shamanic healing. Shamanism is historically, often associated with Earths indigenous and tribal societies and has persisted all over your world since its inception in ancient native cultures. Some of these are Siberian, Indian, Native American, South American and aboriginals. It involves beliefs that shamans, with a connection to the otherworld, have the power to heal the sick, communicate with ethereal light beings, and escort ethereal human essences of the dead to the afterlife. Some of the holistic healing practices of your modern world have been developed from this ancient practice.

To be honest with you Shamanic healing is another book in itself. I will enlighten you on other forms of healing used more in the western modern world, but remember what ever healing you are guided to, TRUST the process, as your celestial guides know what is best for your unique body and mind at the time it is needed.

Some energy healing is hands-on healing where the holistic healer channels a wonderful high source of unconditional love energy. This can be with the hands physically placed on the human body or held in the ethereal human energy field. The celestial guides of both human parties involved work with the healer to send the healing through the recipient's body targeting the areas that need healing. In this process they send healing energy in while removing any unwanted darker energy out of the body. Our celestial guides have learnt with humans that different types of energy from their healing realms can help you. This helped them to create different type of healing practices for humanity, a few examples are Angelic healing, Reiki, Massage (e.g.: Indian head massage) and Distance Healing.

All Earth humans have Chakras and Meridian Points, and they were given to the human form to keep it balanced with high divine energies while existing in the three-dimensional energies. All hands-on energy healing uses these body points to balance the human form.

Reiki and Chakras

Chakras are energy points that run through the central core energy system of the human body. They were given to humanity to help balance the human form in the Earth's energy while connected to the high source energies of the universe. They were used in ancient times in energy healing techniques now called Reiki, but the knowledge was lost over the centuries. Our celestial overseers reintroduced this knowledge again in the nineth century through a human called Mikao Usui from Japan, through his life mission he taught the healing Reiki system to over a two thousand humans that spread this ancient knowledge around the world to help humanity.

The chakra system was added to the human ethereal structure in the third Atlantis experiment period of around 50,000 BC. The master off-world celestial scientists felt the male and female humanoids needed an energy centre to link the feminine and masculine energy to the higher pure quantum source and the pure energy of Earth. *(For more information on this knowledge please refer to the book 'The Light within Atlantis').*

There has been confusion among humans of how many chakras there are, but I would like to confirm there are twelve chakras that I will refer to, to help you understand the human physical form and the connection to source.

The chakra system helps keep humans focused on the higher source and are source energy tools in the human body. The first chakra the Earth Star chakra keeps you grounded in the two and three-dimensional matrix, with the body chakras balancing health and mind. The higher, out-of-physical-body chakras starting at chakra nine the higher self Chakra are energy batteries for the connection to the divine source. The celestial beings can tune into the human form and adjust the energies of these chakras; they guide Earth healers to this work to help humanity.

Chakra one – this is the **Earth star chakra**, which sits below the human form in their ethereal light energy. Physical beings on Earth have a unique connection with the Earth life force and to the crystalline matrix grid in the Earth's mineral ore structure. This is the anchor chakra, keeping your energies grounded and helping to balance your body and mind while you are connected to the higher quantum source of creation.

Chakra two – this is the **root chakra**, and it is located at the base of the humanoid spine in the centre of the physical body. The root chakra is a grounding chakra, which helps human individuals stay centred, secure, active, energised, and present in the moment. It also allows healing energy to flow up from the Earth and into the rest of the chakras. It is an important foundation for the seven chakras that are contained within the physical human body energy field. The root chakra also allows the human form to experience safety and security in their life whenever there is spiritual balance.

Chakra three – this is the **sacral chakra** and is based in the human form above the root chakra at the centre of creativity and sexuality. Its function is to deal with issues of relationships and social interaction; this centre is also the dwelling place of the human's true self. The sacral chakra rules abundance, creativity, wellness and joy, and also controls passions, sex and pleasure, and brings the lesson of learning to let go of past emotions.

Chakra four – this is the **solar plexus chakra**; it sits above the sacral chakra and is the power centre which stores energy – a key chakra for all the chakras to function correctly. The solar plexus is the centre of will, and it controls issues from the past as well as ambitions and goals for success in the future. This is the centre of an individual's personality, and its state of balance is directly correlated to their sense of will power, self-acceptance, and their ambition to succeed. This chakra also highlights health issues in the digestion tracks of the body.

Chakra five – this is the **heart chakra**, located in the centre of the human behind the beating heart in a sacred energy space, and is where the emotional inner being, the physical and the soul connection meet. The heart chakra controls the energy around relationships, and when the chakra is fully open, it allows the love energy to flow through the human being allowing them to relate to others with love and compassion. The heart chakra also allows individuals to be empathetic to the feelings and emotions of others, while remaining true and in tune with their own energy and self. The human heart spiritual base is designed for the heart chakra to help with emotional healing, with love for self and others, as well as overseeing self-appreciation of beauty, and willingness for compassion. The heart chakra is a sacred portal, which gives access to the gifts of your higher energetic centres and is the doorway to the realms to source, knowledge, and divine unconditional love energy.

Chakra six – this is the **throat chakra** and is the human being's communication centre. It is the centre of truth, personal expression, listening, responsibility, facing retribution, faith, and creativity. The way the voice is used is overseen by the throat chakra, through singing, communicating, talking, and listening. When opened and balanced, the throat chakra allows humans to speak their truth of their divine love purpose.

Chakra seven – this is the **third eye chakra** and is located in the centre of the human forehead and links with the penal gland area of the brain. It is the centre of psychic ability and also plays a role in feeling, sensing, and hearing connections to all in the universe. This chakra also connects human energies to beyond the physical form, linking individuals with the subconscious mind and the higher realms of high ascension energy. The third eye chakra oversees learning, memory, telepathy, clairvoyance, channelling, light worker communicator and aura sensing.

Chakra eight – this is the **crown chakra** and is on the crown of the head, connecting the human being to the higher quantum dimensional realms through the higher chakras. When it is awakened it connects to the mind's dreams, imagination, visions, hopes, spiritual downloads, and alignment with their higher self-purpose. When the crown chakra is fully open, humans are linked to the unconditional love of the universal quantum source, which then opens up new knowledge to bring all possibilities in their Earth lifetime. With a lot of humans they shut down from the quantum source after birth, the crown chakra closes. The crown chakra will start to reopen when the human has the spark of unconditional love and higher ascended understanding.

Chakra nine – this is the **higher self chakra**. Chakras nine to twelve sit in line with the other chakras above the human form. When these are activated, it allows the quantum divine light to flow through this energetic centre to access higher consciousness. It travels to the quantum source and then back down to the ethereal light body, chakras, and physical body to replenish, empowering and enlightening. It gives access to unconditional love which can be truly felt and experienced, bringing awareness of the power of the soul within the physical form, enabling spiritual being to be recognised. The higher self chakra acts as a flowing river of soul energy and contains the accumulated soul experiences that can be accessed for divine purpose. When you connect fully to this chakra you find your life mission and your intuition is heightened to help guide you during your journey on Earth.

Chakra ten – this is the **ethereal light body chakra** and when fully opened, will allow the human being to link to the expansive quantum realms of highly ascended beings. It celestial guides them to remember their direct connection with the quantum source, and their ability to communicate with celestial light beings, that you know as angels, celestial guides, and star beings from around the universe. When this chakra is activated, the human willingly surrenders to the flow of the higher dimensional energy. This allows the quantum domains source of creative intelligence to flow into the human experience of existence to help in interpreting telepathically channelled messages. This enables the full extent of the ethereal light bodies connection abilities to be accessed, along with the realisation of their expansive ability to create, which is empowered through the direct connection to the quantum source.

Chakra eleven – this is the **universal chakra** and represents all that exists in the universal quantum energy flow. This chakra is also the access point to the doorway that opens the infinite flow of creation. When this chakra is activated, the human feels in close alignment to the quantum universe and all that is. It also allows for their quantum ethereal light body to be fully constructed, the multi-dimensional transitional being. This then allows unlimited access to travel within the higher realms and dimensions. This can be through thought, dreams, or meditation state of mind to the Astral Earth fourth dimensional plane of existence.

Chakra twelve – this is the **galactic chakra** and is the frequency to the light portals that travel beyond the limits of restrictive time and space, teleportation, instant manifestation, and bi-location, the ability to be in more than two places at a time. When connected, the activated human can reach anywhere in the realms of quantum creation, communicating with the highest vibration celestial beings and ascended masters, including the quantum womb of creation. This also activates healing, insight, and growth from the highest light realms into their existence.

The chakras nine to twelve will be fully activated when the stages of Deep Core Healing are completed. A pure connection to the celestial beings and the quantum domains creative intelligence knowledge depends on this factor. Most light workers will function from chakra one to eight open but can struggle with their connection to the quantum source as its not constant clear information. This is because they are in the 3D/4D reality and their energy dips through, ill health, not trusting the ascension progress existing in fear. The information you need lies in your inner self soul energy and with your higher self and your outer communicators your celestial guides. Trust, heal and you will tap into this knowledge. Reiki healing will help all humans including light workers to heal and a tune to the higher vibration energy of love.

There are further energy points above you and below you that are anchors to the different realities of existence. These are attached to your Earth lifeline to the higher source that can be understood by the human mind eye as a silver thread. This thread is your guiding route back to your source of existence that you originated from.

If you take the time, you can see the link between the twelve chakras and the twelve dimensions explained in this book. Everything is inter-connected, and the chakras were designed to link with these higher energy sources when activated. For the human being to be in a high state of vibrational frequency and stay connected to the unconditional love divine light quantum source, all twelve chakras must be activated. If their energy drops the chakras will start to waver, but healing can regenerate them. If the human form drops into a lower energy, the chakras nine to twelve will shut down, breaking the source link. The crown chakra and third eye chakra will also shut, leaving the other chakras to function in the physical body form alone. The rest of the open chakras will then become under-energised, and the human body will then experience disease and pain.

Meridian Points

The meridian system is a concept re-introduced to humanity through traditional Chinese medicine around three thousand years ago. It has been in our knowledge since humans existed and many other similar celestial species have them and they also work with the meridian energy lines to aid healing in the physical form. This knowledge was passed on to Earth humans in ancient times. They are unseen energy points that help the left and right side of the body work in unison and help balance the human structure. As they are unseen human scientists do not recognise these healing systems because they can't see them. If the doubting human could only think out of the box, and take time to know their own human form, their hands and sixth sense will feel and see the energy system of the human form.

Meridians are used in the practice of acupuncture in the eastern world and has spread to the western world of Earth. Pressure is placed on the meridian points to ease pressure for the energy flow of the body. Meridians are paths through which the life-energy known as "qi" (ch'i) flows – the quantum energy of the universe. A blockage in a meridian is like unplugging two connecting wires that causes an interruption in the flow of energy. The energy will try to reroute itself through other meridians, but this will lead to a buildup of energy on one side of the blockage and a deficiency of energy on the other causing human health issues.

Acupuncture, is one of the primary methods of treatment in traditional oriental medicine, is based on a system of meridians. There are about 400 acupuncture points most of which are situated along 12 primary and eight extraordinary channels. There are "12 Principal Meridians" where each meridian corresponds to either a hollow or solid organ, interacting with it and extending along a particular extremity example an arm or leg. There are also eight extraordinary channels, two of which have their own sets of points, and the remaining ones connecting points on other channels. Along the meridians lie acupuncture points or acupoints, which are stimulated by needling, pressure, or heat to resolve a clinical problem.

Humans were guided to a number of methods to identify meridians and to explain them anatomically - regions of increased temperature and low skin resistance have been suggested to represent meridians or as methods to identify them. Meridians are entities within the body that, when stimulated by acupuncture can result in health improvement.

As with all healing it clears the darker energy sitting in the human form some of this being emotions. This leaves the body through the eyes, pores, nose, mouth or the bladder and bowels. If you experience this after healing, you might feel out of sorts for a couple of days. But trust it will be a big shift for you and your energies for the better so bear with it.

So Reiki chakras healing, and Meridian healing is two methods you can use to keep balanced and help you on your spiritual journey of ascension. Our celestial guides bring this to many lightworkers for their vocation of healing. Or they guide humans that have excepted they need to change and embrace holistic healing instead of clinical drugs as a way to heal.

Angelic Healing

Angelic Healing comes from the source of the twelve celestial Ray light beings we mentioned in the dimensional levels that are connected with the twelve dimensions. Alongside these celestial beings are other light beings that also help with this healing for humanity. Humanity over time came to know them as Angels, for example Archangel Michael or Raphael. To help you identify with these beings they bought themselves to you in the reflection of the human form. Archangels meaning is a high-ranking celestial form sometimes represented to you as an ascended master of their existence.

Humans have been guided over time to create different forms of angelic healing and names for it, including angelic reiki, quantum angel healing, divine universal healing, and angelic ayurveda. This is because humans interpret the angelic energy in their own Earth perspective and the energy can be adjusted by our celestial guides into different frequencies in the different named methods of healing. The basic understanding of each healing method varying but the healing source is from our twelve celestial beings and their helpers.

Many light workers will have an angelic guide as a healer. As many also have a native American guide from the ancient shamanic understanding of the healing source. As with all healing you will need more than one session, but you will be guided by the holistic healer and your celestial guides through your intuition to what you need.

Distant Healing

Distance healing is when a human connects to the universal quantum source, the twelve Ray celestial healing beings and their own celestial guide team and ask for healing to be sent to a human, animal, situation, or place. This is a telepathic link request from your conscious mind that is sent out to the universe where your celestial guides and quantum healing sources will pick up your energy signal and respond. You must recognise this is also the prayer energy humanity has used since they recognised a God source existence in the universe, *The Quantum Domain*. Prayers are often for self, but the ones that are requested to help others with pure intention from the human heart are a more powerful energy source and a stronger signal.

A pure of heart distant healing request will always be heard and answered. But the healing will be delivered in a way that is right for the human, animal, the situation, and place at that time. Remember there is a bigger picture and sometimes events need to play out in a certain way for the spiritual life lessons to be learned for all parties involved.

Often a healing request is sudden of the back of human emotion, and this is a powerful emotion. If you wish to send healing daily as many light workers do, take time to sit in a quite space you feel safe in. Write down who and what needs healing and involve this list in your healing prayer and thoughts. This also is a lovely way to end your human day. Give thanks for all you have, ask for healing for yourself and loved ones and the world as a whole in your distant healing thoughts.

Do you realise that the power of the human mind is an amazing source of energy. Our future is the source of mind healing as well as hands on healing. You will rediscover the power of the pyramid energy source and with your conscious minds you will heal each other and our planet through this amazing energy source. This ancient knowledge is not new to Earth. Our future is community living with healing centres. Humanity will evolve and there will be those among you that will exist to give this healing daily to your planet and humanity.

(In our meditation chapter we have a Pyramid meditation that connects you with the twelve celestial Ray beings and brings you downloads for healing and knowledge).

Sound Healing

Sound healing works with the harmonic sound vibration frequencies that can heal the body's energy from physical cells to the etheric light energy field. Many are being guided in this awakening period to learn about sound healing and being guided to bring sound healing to humanity. The two popular sound healing forms in our modern day is crystal bowls and sound tuning forks. Our scientist of our world is now working with sound vibration. For example it has been used to treat forms of prostate cancers, break up kidney stones and detecting cancer cells. Sound healing is a natural way to treat pain and illness, is simple to use and has no harmful side effects.

Also musical sound vibration can change your mood and distress you, Work with music is being used to help humans with dementia. Also human studies have shown that removing the stress frequencies in a person's voice can reduce high blood pressure and speed up the body's healing process, and that listening to slow rhythms can lower heart rate and decrease stress levels.

This is the future for humanity and changing its perspective on healing in our world. All of this light healing will raise the frequency of peace and unity on Earth. Through sound healing our celestial overseer's mission is to bring the authentic truth to create unity amongst humanity.

Massage

Massage has been a hands-on healing process for the aid of relaxation by massaging the muscles and skin of the human body to release tension for a long time on Earth. The process uses aromatherapy oils that the massager is guided to use. The oils themselves, have various healing properties, remember Mother Nature has all you need to heal the human form if you look after her.

The massage process releases negative energy held in the body that can be released in an emotional way such as tears. It's ancient form of relaxation for easing tension and stress. As with all healing processes it could release the heavier energies through your through the eyes, pores, nose, mouth or the bladder and bowels.

Some of the forms of massage you might be led to on your healing journey are: Indian head massage, Hot stone massage, Aromatherapy massage, Deep tissue massage, Trigger point massage, Reflexology and Shiatsu massage. There are couple of examples below for your knowledge.

Reflexology

Reflexology is a type of massage that involves applying different amounts of pressure to the feet, hands, and ears. There are meridian points on the feet that correspond to organs and systems of the body. Pressure applied to the foot brings relaxation and healing to the corresponding area of the body.

Reflexology can reduce stress, anxiety, pain, lift your mood and general well-being in physical body and mind. The points of connection in the feet link with nerve endings in the body that are linked to organs and muscles including the brain.

Indian Head Massage

Indian head massage is an ancient healing system, and it was gifted to the holy men from the Himalayan region of India around 1800BC Earth time. It is a natural and holistic reproach to physical and mental health. It was derived from the Ayurvedic medicine which is one of the world's oldest medical systems and remains one of India's traditional health care systems in this modern human day.

Indian head massage treatment uses massage movements to help ease muscle strain and tension, while the pressure on various points of the head and neck works the body meridian lines to give treatment to the entire body.

Many find this treatment works well alongside reflexology. It allows the celestial guides through the human healers to work on all regions of the human form from different starting points.

Human Mind Therapy's

Meditation

Meditation is key to any humans, Deep Core Healing and ascension development, as it helps calm the mind opening up clear communication channels to hear or see us.

The Earth word meditation is derived from two Latin words: meditari (to think, to dwell upon, to exercise the mind) and mederi (to heal). Its Sanskrit derivation 'medha' means wisdom, which we feel sums up the word meditation well in our language.

With the hectic pace and demands of our modern Earth life's, many people feel stressed and over-worked. It often feels like there is just not enough time in the Earth day to get everything done. Your stress and tiredness make you unhappy, impatient, and frustrated and it can affect your health. You are often so busy you feel there is no time to stop and meditate! But meditation actually gives you more time by making your mind calmer and more focused. You will learn to put first what is important in life, and as you destress everyday tasks will become easier.

Meditation can also help you to understand our own mind. You learn how to transform your mind from negative thoughts to positive thoughts, from disturbed to peaceful, from unhappy to happy. This will help you analyse your life better and help you keep a truth perception.

In meditation, you are shifting your awareness from the usual focus, of past and future to the now moment creating calmness in the mind. In daily activity, the mind is engaged in observing, discriminating, deciding, analysing and accomplishing. Meditation gives you the opportunity to shift gears, let go of this focus and experience a more peaceful, silent state of being. This in turn helps bring balance to the physical body and mind healing your body cells and energy blocks. Meditation is a must running alongside other methods of healing we have mentioned. For humanity to achieve the ascension level required with Deep Core Healing from a younger age it is **recommend every child is introduced to meditation**. This should be from a very young age as a daily practice. My how our world would evolve in the light this would create.

Different Types of Meditation

The aim of any meditation is to create a relaxed state of body and mind; the mind is awake but calm. Have you heard of the Earth scientific terms of alpha and beta brain levels? Beta is when you are fully awake, making decisions, focusing on past, present and future and using up energy. In the physical beta state, the blood is pumping hard to all vital organs using high energy.

Alpha is the relaxed brain state, but you are not a sleep. Imagine as you get in to bed and you have washed your sheets and they smell fresh and clean. You snuggle down and relax, but awake, that's the calm feeling you need to reach. In alpha state the blood flow as the body relaxes goes more to the outer shell than the inner body.

You want to achieve this meditative state of being in the moment, relaxed and destressed. When stressed you produce a hormone that you can get addicted to, becomes a cycle of a way of being and your body if it has any physical weaknesses will react to stress through these manifesting themselves more tenfold. Good mental state, calmness and focus all helps the physical well-being as well as the mind.

Remember meditation does not have to be complex. Key to successful meditation is finding which one that suits you. There are a few different ways you can meditate listed below:

- With music – guided with a voice and music

- Mantra meditation

- Movement meditation

- On the spot meditation – Mindfulness

Meditation with Voice and Music

Our celestial guides have found observing the human mind that a lot of us when starting meditation will find listening to a guided meditation works best for you to start with. Start off with one that is for relaxation and help you to distress. Then when you are feeling more confident with this form of meditation, try more spiritual meditations for example I mean, linking you with your celestial guides and helping your spiritual connection for example for healing.

As with all meditation samples here they work by distracting you from your daily thoughts and help you to calm your mind. It is key to find meditations that you are comfortable with. This is because you all have individual energy frequencies, and the vibration of sound affects you differently individuals. So finding the right type of tone from music or the spoken voice and the intention of the meditation is vital to success on the meditation journey.

Mantra Meditation

In mantra meditations, you repeat a particular sound or short phrase again and again. This can be done out loud (chanting) or in your mind. It is key you pick a mantra that has spiritual meaning on your path currently and then later changes in intervals as you grow. Repeating words with positive vibration and positive uplifting intention helps to recondition you mind and self-belief of who you are and what you can achieve. This leads to clarity in your thinking and will help you be on a higher vibration, and this helps us work with you telepathically, to bring you guidance and messages.

Using a mantra affirmation while you're meditating helps suppress the thoughts and distractions that arise and gives you a tool to use when you're not meditating. Repeating a meditation mantra during times of stress, for many people, brings about some relaxation and helps them to better deal with whatever the crisis of the moment is. Depending on your belief system, the mantras may also do things like get you in touch with the true nature of the quantum universe, help you spiritually and activate energy centres in the body.

Remember your thoughts are energy and when you do this type of meditation you need to believe what you are repeating and keep in the positive energy mind frame. So as you let doubt come into it, it affects the energy and how the mantra will work. You can ask your celestial guides, spiritual teacher, or meditation teacher to help guide you to the write manta for you at your point in your spiritual journey.

When you could pick your mantra – it could be a simple word like "relax," "serene" "love" or "peace," or something more spiritual like "ohm" or "so-hum" (ancient Sanskrit words meaning "nothingness" and "I am that").

Assume a comfortable but alert upright position and spend 30 seconds just sitting with your eyes closed before starting your mantra breathing steadily. As effortlessly and silently as possible, begin repeating your mantra to yourself (not aloud), over and over. A good method is to get into a smooth breathing pattern, with the words being said in your head on the outward breath. If your mind wanders, just observe the thought, let it pass by and go back to repeating the mantra. The more you practice, the easier this will become for you. There's no need to try to change or stop your thoughts in anyway – just keep whispering the word(s) silently to yourself. The repetition of a mantra quiets the breath and as a result the mind, guiding you into the field of *"Pure Consciousness."* From a beginner's perspective, using a mantra can help focus and sharpen a mind prone to wandering during meditation. As our channeler friend does, if you are on your own while doing this ask us to stop you after 15 minutes. Then just bring yourself back into your space and sit for a bit reflecting on how you feel.

You can do one-word mantras or try something longer. A few suggestions of present tense affirmations for you:

My mind is clear and focused

My body is relaxed and calm

I am at peace within myself

I am focused on the present moment

A few suggestions for Future Tense Affirmations you:

My mind is becoming quiet and relaxed

I will release all stress and tension

I am finding it easier to detach from my thoughts

I will let go of all worries

A few suggestions for Natural Affirmations you:

My mind is naturally calm and tranquil

I have a peaceful mind

Mental serenity is mine

I can let go of my thoughts at will

The 'I am' moments

I would also suggest what I call the **'I am'** affirmations, to become aware of self and raise your energies this way.

The **'I am'** moment is key to you lifting your energies; remember this all starts with you. I suggest you do an 'I am' meditation mantra for five minutes each day when you awake, repeating the chosen affirmation to reinforce the positive energy vein in your lives. I have listed a few below for you to try:

I am Love and joy

I am happy

I am willing to let go

I am the best I can be

I am beautiful

I am loved

I am strong and powerful

I am calm

I am at peace

I am loved

I am well and healthy

Meditation Through Body Movement

Qigong practice typically involves moving meditation, coordinating slow-flowing movement, deep rhythmic breathing, and a calm meditative state of mind. People practice qigong throughout China and worldwide for recreation, exercise, relaxation, preventive medicine, self-healing, alternative meditation, self-cultivation, and training for martial arts.

Yoga practice is a mind and body practice. Various styles of yoga combines physical postures, breathing techniques and meditation or relaxation. Yoga is an ancient process that promotes mental and physical well-being.

Mindfulness - On the Spot Meditations

I know this is a positive way forward for humanity to help you connect more with yourself, the world around you and us. Learning and understanding mindfulness will also aid you in meditation, which helps to destress you, clearing and raising your energies to aid ascension in the energy levels.

The benefits of mindfulness help in these ways:

1. It cultivates more awareness and stabilises the mind

2. You become clear seeing (have clarity) in everything around you and within yourself

3. It changes your perspective on your world and your thought patterns

4. It brings wisdom, as you see your world differently

5. It helps destress you by casting worrying thoughts to the side and giving your busy mind a rest.

Our minds are amazing things, with great power that could unfold great things for you as an individual. At the moment our minds are restricted by dwelling on our past memories and emotions, which then influence how you look at your future. Your mind is judgmental and creates its own miss-perceptions of situations and the world around you.

Your mind connects to your senses - sight, hearing, touch, smell and taste. Our celestial guides see us live our lives without seeing, hear without hearing, touch without touching, smell without smelling and taste without truly tasting. You also have another sense, **Knowing**, which is like a sixth sense and is in your mind field and your light energy field. *What do I mean?* Knowing is something that you use without realising it, but it is a weak sense at the moment in most of you. When tapped into and strengthened, this ability will bring you knowledge from the universe, clarity to your thinking, wisdom, and greater understanding. And very importantly it helps with your development as a light worker channeler and strengthens your connection to your celestial guides. This is because when your mind is less busy, they can connect telepathically to you better. Also this will help a light worker channeller learn to have a less busy mind when giving messages and focus on the clear ethereal essence energy thoughts and images coming in.

You rush along in your world, thinking you are aware of the world around you, but you are not. The simplest way for me to describe this in words is to give an example: You are given ten red pencils laid out next to each other in a row; most people will think they are all the same and not take a second look at them as long as they function and serve the purpose that is all that matters. BUT each pencil is unique! If you stopped and looked at each individual pencil, you would be able to describe each one and the uniqueness that makes them different from each other. As you did this you would be more aware of that moment in time, as if you have slowed down time to stop and become aware of these 10 red pencils. You can feel them, look at them all over, smell them, listen to them, and even taste them. When you are this aware you are being **mindful, and this is what mindfulness means**.

I do laugh though, I say be more aware, but if you followed this example of the red pencils to everything in your day, you would not get much done! *BUT do you see what I am saying?*

Holistic Emotion Healing

This is a method of energy releasing is done through the twelve celestial Ray beings working with the light worker channeler or holistic healer and the recipient of the healing.

It sets the intention to release any memories that holds negative emotion with them. It will allow the memory to stay but without the emotion attached to it that is holding the human back on their spiritual path. Remember negatives energies are of a low vibration so when it is removed it raises your vibration and outlook on life.

This method is done through the light worker channeler or holistic healer talking to the recipient into a meditate calm state to meditation music. The recipient lies down in a calm room where they won't be disturbed. The light worker before they start asks the recipient to decide on the one memory they wish to work on and during the meditation they release the trauma around this memory over to the twelve celestial beings. I have included in the meditation chapter of the book a meditation that takes you through this process which is **key for Deep Core Healing** to be successful.

NLP, Counselling, and Holistic Therapies

I have asked my friend **Human B** to explain to us their experience of NLP for this wonderful book. I feel it is good for your understanding to get a real human perspective on this subject.

Human B: In my experience what do I think is the difference between counselling and NLP?

From experience I find that counselling and NLP have different purposes depending on each individual and how you want to seek guidance and assistance.

From a personal perspective, I find counselling more helpful as a talking therapy when you want to offload through speaking and being heard. I'll generally go for counselling when I would rather off load the things that I have gone through with a professional who has an outside point of view, who isn't inside the emotions with you and has a fresh perspective to share. I look at both counselling and NLP as personal development which takes the stigma away.

Counselling works with the conscious part of your mind, meaning, you are working in the now with the part of your brain that is aware and learning in the moment.

NLP (Neuro Linguistic Programming) works with the unconscious part of the mind and stands for:

- **Neuro** - Neurological pathways, unconscious mind, conscious mind, nervous system (carries electrical messages to and from the brain, connecting to the body and soul) through external experiences of the senses: Visual, Auditory, Kinesthetic, Olfactory, Gustatory (site, sound, touch, smell, taste).
- **Linguistic** - Language, how you communicate non-verbally in which our brains process through, pictures, sounds, feelings, tastes, smells, words as in how you speak to yourself inside your mind, all put together to represent and give meaning.
- **Programming** - How we communicate with ourselves and others from learnt behaviors, patterns, beliefs, values, memories, strategies, attitude etc. that is running in the background in our UNCONSCIOUS

MIND (e.g. things that run in the background such as breathing).

In other words, NLP works and deals with the core issue, builds on top of what you already know, can be content free (meaning you don't have to keep repeating and speaking about something in order for it to work). For example, you can change a limiting belief that has been holding you back for years in around 20 minutes.

Changes happen quicker with NLP than counselling. I do believe that both counselling and NLP have their place in people's lives at the right time and place, depending on where they are on their life's path.

Both NLP and counselling can be solution based, meaning that both seek to work towards an end goal that someone has in mind. NLP tends to last longer than counselling because you're working with the unconscious part of the mind, which is 95% of your mind's capacity, whereas the conscious part of your mind is only 5%! All your habits, beliefs, language, attitude, programming (things learnt from others as you grow up from a young age), memories, space, matter, and energy are stored in the unconscious part of the mind. In my personal opinion this is another reason why NLP is so effective compared to counselling in making changes at a core level.

In NLP through the communication model, we're taught that events that happen outside of us come into our senses such as, touch, sight, taste, smell, sound and I've added EMF (electromagnetic field – aura). The unconscious mind will then, delete distort or generalise what is going on for you into smaller chunks of info. This then gives you your unique inner point of view of the world (your model of the world), which creates our state of mind, how our bodies react (physiology) which then creates our behaviours (what we do). As shown below:

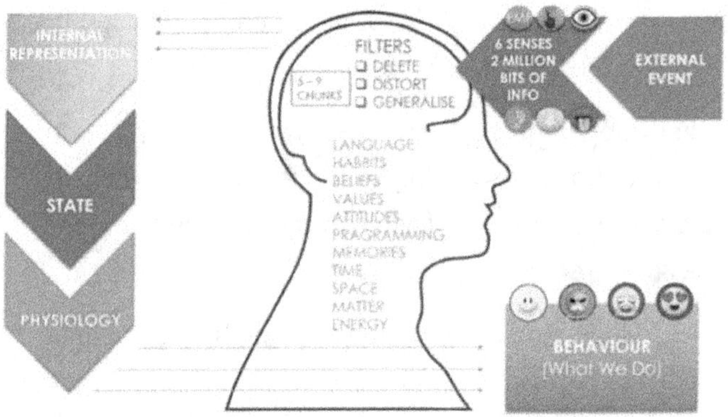

Picture credit to Amanda Bowden – Transitional Coach

I am trained up to counselling level two but have experienced working with CBT, which stands for, cognitive behavioural therapy. Basically, working with your thoughts, feeling and behaviours.

In CBT, the pattern can be seen using a circle where a thought can lead to feeling emotions which can lead to a behaviour (something you do through action). But this can happen and start at any stage on the picture opposite.

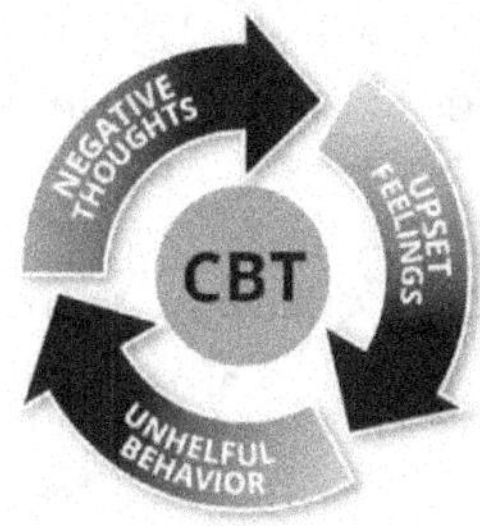

In my experience, it's taken less time using NLP to make changes than counselling.

Time Line Therapy is a technique that takes the positive learnings from past memories unconsciously and helps to let go of what we call *"THE BIG 5"* negative emotions of:

- ✓ Anger
- ✓ Sadness
- ✓ Fear
- ✓ Hurt
- ✓ Guilt

and all the subset negative emotions that fall under these emotions.

Time Line Therapy is content free, quick, effective and comfortable.

Time Line Therapy helps you to let go of repressed negative emotions that can harm the body causing stress and disease (emotions that are felt in the body are called somatics).

Time Line Therapy helps to bring clarity around limiting decisions and limiting beliefs that prevent success in life.

Time Line Therapy helps you to move forward and develop new positive strategies for coping, motivation for life and a more compelling life.

It's one of the best techniques and has had one of the biggest impacts on myself and others who I have worked with.

Hypnosis also works with the unconscious part of your mind. It's nothing like you see on T.V. or the movies. It helps you to feel relaxed a bit like the feeling you get when you're daydreaming, in between dream state and waking up or you can also relate to the feeling that you get if you work with your celestial guides in trance.

Hypnosis is amazing for making quick and effective changes by talking to the unconscious part of the mind through positive suggestions. With relaxing music quietly in the background hypnosis can help with building confidence, manifesting, letting go of negative emotions stored in the body, pretty much anything that you want to solve an issue but at the same time, want to have some me time to sit back and relax.

Some of my favourite techniques that have had the most impact is:

- Hypnotherapy
- Time line Therapy™
- Parts Integration – Brings battling thoughts in your mind together to work in harmony and synergy

NLP is a psychotherapy yet is also classed as a holistic therapy due to how unique it is.

There are many types of counselling, but CBT is one of the easiest and most basic to use and work with.

NLP has not yet been recognised by the NHS even though it has amazing results and gets to the core of problems whereas, CBT is recognised by the NHS, is one of the least effective long term but is cheaper to fund.

If you go through the NHS for a counselling service, you will generally be offered only 6 sessions with a counsellor which is not always long enough when doing conscious work. The waiting times are generally quite high, even more so now in 2022 than the past due to ongoing events in our world.

How Hypnotherapy Supports Inner Deep Core Healing

Hypnotherapy along with Quantum Trance Healing is one of the most effective bridges between the conscious mind, the subconscious mind, and the ethereal energy body. Because Deep Core Healing requires the release of trauma, outdated beliefs, and emotional imprints held deep within the human essence, hypnotherapy can support this journey in profound and accelerated ways. It works by guiding you into a deeply relaxed state where the layers of the subconscious become accessible. This is where the emotional residue of old experiences, fear, limitation, conditioning, and unconscious programming, has been stored. Through this gentle access, hypnotherapy helps uncover and dissolve the inner blocks that the human mind cannot reach on its own.

Much of the trauma and emotional density you carry is not only psychological, but it also embeds itself into the ethereal energy body. These blockages often interfere with intuition, spiritual perception, emotional clarity, and vitality. Hypnotherapy softens and loosens this energetic residue. When the nervous system relaxes, the energy field expands, creating an opening for your ethereal light self, your celestial guides, and your higher self to assist in deeper healing. As this density clears, you experience greater clarity and alignment with your soul plan.

Deep Core Healing requires a shift in consciousness, and hypnotherapy supports this by gently reprogramming the mind. Old stories of fear, rejection, and limitation are replaced with narratives rooted in self-love, personal truth, and higher awareness. This mental shift is essential, because healing cannot be sustained if the mind remains aligned with outdated patterns. Hypnotherapy creates new inner pathways, supporting confidence, emotional balance, and spiritual receptivity.

One of the most powerful aspects of hypnotherapy is the way it strengthens your connection to your higher self. When the conscious mind becomes quiet, higher knowing rises naturally to the surface. Many people receive vision-like impressions, deep intuitive messages, or soul plan level insights that clarify their purpose. This inner communication becomes easier and more consistent over time, enhancing spiritual development.

The physical body also responds positively to hypnotherapy. Emotions directly influence the body's chemistry and tension patterns. By helping you release inner stress, hypnotherapy supports immune function, calms the nervous system, and reduces the physical symptoms that come from emotional and spiritual imbalance. When emotional layers heal, the body begins to repair itself more naturally.

Finally, hypnotherapy deepens your connection with your celestial guides. In a relaxed state, the human mind becomes more open to subtle frequencies, enabling you to sense your guides' presence, receive impressions, and develop trust in their communication. Many experience colours, sensations, or subtle guidance that feels more vivid and accessible.

In essence, hypnotherapy is both a psychological tool and a spiritual doorway. It supports Deep Core Healing by opening the subconscious, clearing old energy, repairing the emotional landscape, strengthening the higher-self connection, and allowing the body to heal from the inside out. Through this work, you become aligned with your soul plans blueprint and more prepared for the ascension journey ahead. One of the most effective bridges between the conscious mind, the subconscious mind, and the ethereal energy body.

Quantum Trance Healing

Quantum Trance Healing supports Deep Core Healing by allowing humans to access the multi-dimensional layers of their existence, far beyond the limitations of the present lifetime. When a person enters the quantum trance state, the mind shifts from linear awareness into a non-linear field where past, present, and future time lines exist simultaneously. This expanded awareness enables old trauma, karmic residue, and emotional imprints from past lives to rise to the surface so they can be released from the deep core of the energy body. These unresolved energies often influence human behaviour, emotional reactions, and physical health without conscious understanding. In the quantum state, they become visible, understood, and finally cleared.

At the same time, Quantum Trance Healing also connects the human to future time lines versions of themselves already aligned with higher consciousness, emotional freedom, and spiritual expansion. These future aspects carry codes of healing, clarity, and empowerment that can be brought back into the present self. This *"future-self integration"* is a powerful catalyst for Deep Core Healing, because it allows the human to embody the vibration of who they are becoming rather than repeating the suffering of who they once were.

One of the most profound gifts of Quantum Trance Healing is the restoration of the ethereal light body. This light body holds the memory of your true essence unconditional, limitless, and whole. Throughout human life, the ethereal body becomes weighed down by grief, fear, stress, and accumulated energetic debris. In the quantum state, celestial guides work directly on this body, repairing tears, clearing dense energies, and rebalancing the frequency fields that feed into the physical body. When the light body heals, the physical and emotional self follow naturally.

This healing also brings you into deeper alignment with your soul plan, the blueprint created before Ethereal Connection to the physical form. Quantum trance opens communication between the human consciousness and the higher self, allowing you to understand why certain experiences were chosen and what lessons are unfolding. This understanding dissolves resistance, fear, and confusion, replacing them with acceptance and clarity. When you reconnect with your soul plan, your life begins to flow with more purpose, intuition, and synchronicity.

Finally, Quantum Trance Healing strengthens the bond with your higher self, allowing a merging of human awareness with divine wisdom. The higher self with the trance guides becomes the guide, the healer, and the steady anchor throughout the process. This alignment accelerates Deep Core Healing by helping you see life through a higher perspective, freeing you from old identities, and guiding you toward emotional liberation and spiritual evolution. Through this multi-dimensional work, Quantum Trance Healing truly transforms the human from the inside out, healing the past, empowering the present, and activating the future path of the soul plan.

Chapter six

Healing Meditations

Meditation unlocks emotional release, deep peace, and soul plan alignment by allowing the higher self to speak through the quiet mind. This chapter guides you through structured healing meditations for empowerment, grounding, clarity, and transformation.

Meditation is one of the most powerful gateways to emotional release, spiritual growth, and deep inner transformation. In the stillness of the mind, the voice of the ethereal light body quantum connection and higher self can be heard, and the healing frequencies of celestial support can be received without interference. Through guided meditations, humans learn to step out of the thinking mind and into the inner chamber of higher self soul plan wisdom, where healing becomes natural rather than forced.

This chapter introduces structured meditations designed to activate different aspects of your Deep Core Healing journey. Each is encoded with high-frequency light code support to assist emotional clearing, grounding, clarity, and the dissolution of lower energies held within the body and energy field.

The Purpose of Healing Meditation

Meditation has always been a bridge between physical consciousness and higher-dimensional quantum intelligence.

When you enter a meditative state, your brain shifts into a calm and receptive frequency.

Here:

• Your nervous system resets

• Emotional pressure softens

• The busy thinking mind becomes quiet

• Your celestial guides and higher self can transmit insight, memory, healing, and direction.

Meditation makes space for the inner healer to awaken.

In Deep Core Healing, guided meditations are not simply for relaxation, they are active energetic experiences. When you listen with open intention, your celestial guides and the Twelve Ray Celestial Beings connect to your ethereal light body quantum energy field, working directly with your energy system to shift what is ready to be released.

Some meditations work with the chakras, others with memory, others with grounding or higher consciousness, and some with deep emotional cellular clearing. All of them, however, move you forward.

I encourage you to keep a meditation journal to record your experiences. Over time, you will be able to look back and see how each meditation has supported your healing, expanded your awareness, and brought greater clarity to your Deep Core Healing spiritual journey.

How These Meditations Work

My celestial guides have channelled six mediations to help with the Deep Core Healing Process. Each meditation carries its own encoded frequency, similar to a healing *"Key."* When activated through listening or reading, the body and energy field begin releasing emotions, trauma patterns, outdated beliefs, and energetic blockages no longer needed for your evolution.

These healing transmissions operate on multiple layers:

1. **Conscious Mind** – mindfulness, understanding, insight

2. **Subconscious Mind** – memory, emotion, programming

3. **Cellular Body** – physical tension, somatic imprint

4. **Energetic Ethereal Light Body** – Ethereal aura, chakras, meridians points

5. **Higher Self and Soul Plan** – life lessons and karmic patterns

When inner resistance drops, your whole system opens, allowing high-frequency healing energy to flow.

You do not need to *"Try."* You simply need to receive.

Trusting the Process

People often worry that they cannot visualise easily or that their thoughts wander. This is normal. Even if your mind drifts, the healing still works, because you are not doing the healing, your celestial guides and higher self are.

What matters most is:

• Intention

• Willingness

• Consistency

Set a simple intention before beginning:

"I allow myself to receive the highest healing available to me now."

This alone opens the door for the work to take place.

Support from the Higher Realms

When you use these meditations, your celestial guides and the Twelve Ray Celestial Beings connect with you. They provide the frequency needed for your level of awakening, not too much, not too little, but exactly what you are ready to integrate.

As your vibration rises, the same meditation will reveal deeper layers, meaning one recording may serve you dozens of times throughout your journey, each time accessing a different emotional or energetic shift.

Nothing is random.

Nothing is wasted.

Every session moves you forward, even when you feel nothing.

NOTE: *When you engage in these meditation practices, make sure you are in a quiet space with no distractions, do not do them when driving or using machinery. You can ask a friend to read the meditations to you while*

Deep Core Healing Mind and Body Meditation

This meditation has been channeled by my celestial guides
to bring knowledge to you of self-healing for your mind set
and physical body. It is designed to heal and program your
body cells with an unconditional love high frequency energy
through a positive thought process. This ancient way of
healing sits within the conscious layers of your DNA, and this
meditation will awaken this knowledge and set you on the
path of young at heart, healthy and pain free life.

You are born into this 3D reality of Earth, in a high energy
vibrational frequency of unconditional love and you come
with all the ancient spiritual tools you need to survive this
heaver 3D energy world called Earth. But from birth you are
indoctrinated with the heavier energies of centuries of a
belief system that you will age mentally and physically,
suffering illness, disease, and pain. You think you will die as
an old person, probably ill, slow of mind and unwanted and
no use to society and not wanting to be a burden to others.
This deep-set mind pattern creates this as your reality. To
release the ancient tools given to you, you must create a
positive mindset to change your perception and Earth
reality.

We bring you this ancient frequency meditation to use as
part of yourself healing journey and to change your way of
thinking into a positive way of existence. Our Human A has
personally controlled her own ailments of Fibromyalgia and

osteoarthritis with this positive thought process. Her early journey with these two conditions was very debilitating as it affected her physical and mental health. Even to the point she could not walk upstairs well, and every life function was so painful. After years of medication, for pain control and a decent night's sleep, she came to the mind set through her spiritual ascension work to stop taking the medication and visualised herself FREE of it.

She also got control of her drink and food intake and fitness levels and started to live a healthier lifestyle. She has worked hard with her celestial guides to achieve this for herself creating the best version she can be of herself. For humanity to change they need to self-heal and live a life of kindness in love and support of others. They will then ascend releasing themselves from the heavy restrictive 3D energy into the light energies of 4D and 5D existence. This will create a world of no illness and pain.

Using this meditation as part of your healing plan, will keep yourself healthy and most of the time pain FREE.

The principle behind this message is your cells renew and rejuvenate, and you can influence this process. With a positive thought process of full health and long life, believing you will not physically age into a debilitating state of being and staying young at heart we can maintain a healthy physical and mental balance and have a longer healthier life.

This meditation is part of a process you will need to undertake, and to achieve this you need to work at your ascension thought process from your 3D reality of fear and self-doubt to a 5D reality of love. You need to heal your past and any Earth life emotions that stop you fulfilling your Earth life mission and learn to ground yourself while on this journey of ascension. You need to turn your mind set from aggressive hate thoughts to others, to forgiveness, kindness, and consideration. One way you can counteract this negative thought process is by sending unconditional love to those that affect your energy in a negative way through their actions. You need to learn to love yourself to eliminate self-doubt in your mind and others and trust your spiritual journey of change.

We recommend if you choose to try this self-healing path, if you are on medications, you inform your doctor you are trying to make changes through meditation to improve your health. Then you can work with them to control reduction of medication. We now take you into the healing meditation.

Meditation for Deep Core Healing

Never meditate when driving or using machinery. Always be in a safe space where you can relax and not be disturbed and have a glass of water ready for after the meditation as this will help ground you and refocus your mind.

Now relax and shut your eyes and take your focus to your breathing, take in a deep breath, breathing in the love and light energy now surrounding you and release any worries, fears, and anxiety as you breath out. Take in another a deep breath in, breathing in the love and light energy, *(do this a couple more times).*

I want you to take yourself to somewhere on Earth you have felt your happiest and safe, creating a happy energy space. This can be for example a holiday destination, a view you have loved, your garden or even your own home.

Now I want you to think of someone on Earth you love unconditionally which can be past or present and they can be family, friend, or pet. Take yourself and this person or pet to your happy energy space. Visualise your energies blending together creating an energy field of unconditional love. *(Short pause here).*

Staying in your happy energy space, feeling relaxed, I want you now to scan your body and high light in your mind where you suffer pain or have any weak areas in your physical body and mind.

Now imagine a beautiful pink ball of light pulsating above your head. This high vibrational pink energy of unconditional love starts to flow through your energy portal called the crown chakra on top of your head into your physical body as you do this. The pink energy now travels into your neck, shoulders and down your arms to your fingertips. From the base of your neck down your spine spreading across your back as it travels. It now surrounds your heart centre and organs traveling to your stomach area. You are feeling very relaxed now as this beautiful energy takes hold and moves slowly through your body. This beautiful healing energy now travels to your hips, thighs, knees and calf's, traveling down to your feet. Focus this energy now through your physical body to where the pain is in your body setting the intent it renews your cells, so they are pain free.

As it travels through your body it will clear any negativity and start to repair damaged cells that does not serve your Earth life. Hold this energy in your body sending the love to the parts that give you pain or weakness, setting the intent of no more pain, repeating in your mind 'I deserve a pain free life and I will have a pain free life', repeating again 'I deserve a pain free life and I will have a pain free life'.

Now set the intention to release all this pain over to your healing celestial guides that are with you to take it away.

Now imagine the pink energy expanding out of your body filling your happy energy space. Focus on your thoughts now and say in your mind, 'I am young at heart, healthy and pain free' imagine this wonderful feeling expanding out into your happy energy space. Feel the unconditional love that surrounds you and absorb this into every cell of your body. I am now going to leave you for a while in this beautiful healing energy to enjoy this experience. *(Pause for 10 minutes just playing background music)*.

I ask you now place a hand on your heart and feel this new power within you. This is your own healing power that sits within you at all times. This is the power of positive thought and control over your own reality that creates your destiny.

I ask you to TRUST this new inner powerful connection you have within yourself from the divine source and the universe. It brings you intuition, great strength and is your support system while here on Earth. Building this positive power from within will enhance you Earth life creating a reality of pain free body, clear mind, living with no disease and a life of good health. Remember your thoughts are very powerful and a positive thought pattern and TRUST will keep you linked with this empowerment from within. This inner power is connected to your soul, higher self and divine source of the universe.

Every morning start your day with the manifestation of positive thought 'I am young at heart, healthy and pain free'. When you go to bed at night ask your celestial guides to come round you to give you healing and to always keep you healthy and well. Do this meditation on a regular basis to remind your deep-set consciousness to send the positive high vibration to your body cells so they are always programmed with positive energy.

Focusing on your breath take a deep breath in, becoming more aware of your physical body. Take another deep breath in and wriggle your toes and fingers. Open your eyes and sit for a few minutes and then have some water.

Your body is now rejuvenated, and you have triggered your ancient DNA healing knowledge. From now on with positive mind set you will heal your mindset and physical body.

Take time to reflect on your experience and learn to embrace this new empowerment you have and use it for the good of self and humanity. You must commit to this self-healing path and over time it will become second nature to you and part of your daily life process. Use this meditation regularly to enhance the positivity you need to self-heal and enhance your ascension path here on Earth.

Thank you for participating in this meditation, love, and

blessings to you.

Energy Release Healing Meditation

The meditation is guided for experienced light workers to give the recipient of the healing, healing energy to release unwanted negative energy that's held in the human physical body. We feel this is a meditation is best done with a supporting presence like a healer present to help guide you.

This is a method of energy releasing as we said earlier in the book that is working with the twelve celestial beings who will work with the light worker healer and recipient. These beings might be shown to the light worker and recipient as a human form of Archangel Michael and Archangel Raphael for your comfort. Or you might see colour as they present themselves in colour as explained earlier in the book.

The recipient must set the intention to release any memories that holds negative emotion with them. It will allow the memory to stay but without the emotion attached to it that is holding the human back on their spiritual path. Remember negatives energy are of a low vibration so when removed it raises your vibration and outlook on life. When successful the recipient over time will fell this memory fade into a distant memory energy field. When it is recalled to the surface it will not have the emotional attachment energy, and the recipient will feel slightly detached from it.

The light worker healer needs to before the meditation to talk to the recipient of the healing, asking them to select a memory that needs to heal. They can discuss this memory with the light worker healer or choose to keep it private. Tell the recipient to imagine from their heart center a silver threat attached to a balloon. In this balloon in the meditation, they will place their memory they wish to have healing placed around.

Make it clear to the recipient they must have pure intention to heal this memory so they can advance on their life's ascension journey. Then explain to the recipient to signal they have released the energy by raising the first finger on their dominant hand. If the recipient has not released after 10 minutes guide them back into the room following the meditation. If this happens it means the recipient has not wished to let go of this energy at this time. You must consider they could be thriving of this negative energy and need more understanding of the spiritual journey to release it. Or they need longer in the meditation energy to let go. The light worker will be guided to which scenario it is and repeat the meditation on another occasion when the recipient is ready.

Meditation for Energy release healing

Never meditate when driving or using machinery. Make sure you are in a quite space you will not be disturbed. Have a glass of water ready for after the meditation.

Relax and shut your eyes and take your focus to your breathing, take in a deep breath, breathing in the love and light energy now surrounding you and release any worries, fears and anxiety as you breath out. *(Repeat this twice more.)*

Now imagine a silver threat coming out of your heart center and it has a silver balloon tied on the end of it. Palace in the balloon the memory you wish to have healing placed around.

Now imagine you are standing in a hay field in long grass with wildflowers all around you. The sky is a clear blue, and the sun is high in the sky. It is a warm summers day and there are soft fluffy clouds gently moving a long on the warm summers breeze.

In the distance you see the sea sparkling in the sunshine. You can see a path in front of you leading towards the sea and a beach.

As you approach the beach you can smell the fresh sea air and can feel the soft warm breeze on your skin. A gentle sloping path leads down to the beach. As you step on to the beach you can feel the warm sand between your toes. The sea is gently lapping up on the beach, and you can see the birds soaring on the wind above you.

As you move up the beach in the distance you can see two figures waiting for you. As you approach these two wonderful light celestial beings you can feel the unconditional love, they radiate out to you. As you approach one of the beings will step forward and place some silver scissors in your hand.

They ask you when you are ready to cut with the silver scissors the silver thread letting the balloon go and watch it float away into the blue sky. Please signal with the first finger on your dominant hand when you have released the balloon.

(Play the music for 10 minutes here).

Thank the two celestial beings for their healing and walk slowly back up the beach. Sit down on the sand and breath in the fresh sea air and enjoy the sparkles glinting on the sea in the sun. *(One minute music pause here).*

It is time for your celestial guides to step back who have supported the celestial beings in the healing process, thank your celestial guides for this wonderful experience and the healing you have received.

Now come back slowly to awareness in your quite space, slowly into full Earth consciousness. Take some deep breaths in and wriggle your toes and fingers. Sit there for a few minutes so you can become fully aware of your personal space. Now have a drink of water to help ground you.

Thank you for participating in this wonderful meditation, love, and blessings to you.

Mother Earth's Grounding Meditation

Welcome to our Mother Earth's meditation, we have mentioned grounding already, but this is a guided deeper meditation. This meditation has been channelled from us to help you in your busy human daily life's and when working with the high ascension spirit energy. Use the meditation when you feel you are running on a high vibration energy feeling anxious or after a busy stressful day. Our Human A uses this meditation in her spiritual development groups to help the students settle and balance so they can work with the high ascension spirit beings, while staying grounded to

Mother Earth. We also recommend this meditation to all of humanity to help them develop in meditation and stay grounded.

Never meditate when driving or using machinery. Always be in a safe space where you can relax and not be disturbed and have a glass of water ready for after the meditation.

Meditation for grounding with Mother Earth

Sitting in a supportive chair make sure your feet are on the ground with no shoes. Now relax and shut your eyes and take your focus to your breathing, take in a deep breath, breathing in the love and light energy now surrounding you and release any worries, fears, and anxiety as you breath out. Take in another a deep breath, breathing in the love and light energy, *(do this two more times).*

As you relax you will find yourself being surrounded by a beautiful golden energy from the divine source of unconditional love. This golden energy will gently flow over your body surrounding you. Imagine the energy now flowing into the top of your head through your crown chakra, feel the energy working its way into your muscles as you relax. As it travels through your body it will clear any negative energy that does not serve your Earth life.

The energy now travels into your neck, shoulders and down your arms to your fingertips. From the base of your neck down your spine spreading across your back as it travels. It now surrounds your heart centre and organs traveling to your stomach. You are feeling very relaxed now as this beautiful energy takes hold and moves slowly through your body.

This beautiful healing energy now travels to your hips, thighs, knees, and calf's, traveling down to your feet. As it enters your feet, imagine from the bottom of your feet you are growing golden roots through fresh green grass into Mother Earth.

The roots enter the layers of Mother Earth, traveling through the soil, minerals, and granite layers, through the beautiful crystal layers with amazing colours shining and sparkling. Down and down and down they travel to you reach Mothers Earth's golden core, her beating heart. Mother Earth receives this divine energy and disburses your negative energy with her love.

She is now sending you her healing energy, a beautiful emerald green energy starts to work its way up the roots, through the layers of Mother Earth, the crystal layers, granite layers, minerals and soil, entering though your feet. This healing energy blends with the golden energy as it travels through your body. Imagine it traveling up your calf's, knees, and thighs to your hips. To your stomach, organs, and heart centre, now up from the base of the spine to your neck and from your fingertips to your shoulders. This beautiful healing energy carries on blending with the divine golden energy as it travels to you neck and head leaving though your crown chakra, joining the gold divine healing energy.

Now imagine you are floating in a bubble in a safe space allowing the golden and green energies to merge together, cleansing your aura, The green and gold energy swirls round you, over your head and under your feet. You feel light and relaxed connected with Mother Earth and the divine source, you are now as one with Mother Earth and balanced.

Now take this healing energy that surrounds you into your heart centre where it will stay to keep you grounded and balanced as you walk your Earth's life. Focusing on your breath take a deep breath in, becoming more aware of your physical body. Take another deep breath in and wriggle your toes and fingers. Open your eyes and sit for a few minutes and then have some water.

Thank you for participating in this wonderful grounding meditation, love and blessings to you all.

Pyramid Meditation

This meditation is designed to awaken deep set consciousness in your ancient DNA. As you progress through the meditation it takes you on a journey through twelve levels of ascension linked with the twelve dimensions of our universe. You will be joined by your celestial guides and twelve celestial light beings that have collected to be part of this meditation. They are ancient celestial beings that have served Earth for over twelve thousand years. They come with their energy of light, harmonic sound and colour wave high vibrations, the basis of all creation. Humanity have named them Archangels but show themselves today in their true form of harmonic colour ray vibration to help your next step on your ascension path.

Never meditate when driving or using machinery. Always be in a safe space where you can relax and not be disturbed and have a glass of water ready for after the meditation.

Pyramid meditation - Relax and focus on your breathing. In your imaginations take yourselves to a beautiful oasis, full of fountains of water and beautiful gardens and creatures. In front of you is a golden pyramid. Follow the path in front of you to the entrance to the pyramid where there is a golden door.

Open the door and enter the pyramid though the golden doorway in front of you, you are now on the first dimensional level for humanity.

Level 1 - the consciousness of physical matter – we are joined by the light being Amber Ray – We bring you grounding in this beautiful energy of the Amber Ray. This energy is linked with Mother Earth and the human Earth chakra. Allow the Amber ray light to pass through your crown chakra on the top of your head through your central body and chakras to your Earth chakra that rests below your feet, and this will be anchoring you to Mother Earth. The Amber Ray energy will keep you balanced through this meditation. Now go to the steps in the far-right corner of this sacred space that leads to the next level. Climb the 12 steps as I count with you, 1, 2, 3, 4, 5, 6, 7, 8, 9, 10, 11, 12, you are now on the next level.

Level 2 - the consciousness of elemental frequencies - we are joined by the light being Emerald Ray – We bring you Emerald Ray's energy from the trees, animals and insects on your Earth. Imagine you are standing in a forest and can feel the ancient strength of the forest around as you stand in the calmness of nature, let her healing energy heal you, imagine you are breathing in the smell of Mother Earth scents to bring a stronger connection to her. Focus and hold this energy in your heart. Now go to the steps in the far-right corner of this sacred space that leads to the next level. Climb the 12 steps as I count with you, 1, 2, 3, 4, 5, 6, 7, 8, 9, 10, 11, 12, you are now on the next level.

Level 3 - the consciousness of the conscious being – we are joined by the light being Fire Red Ray – The energy of Fire Red Ray brings you a warrior's courage to deal with the challenging 3D energy matrix on Earth. The energy brings you balance to deal with old emotions and new life experiences. We now want you to set the intent to heal your pass so you can move forward on your Earth's path. Look deep into your heart centre and hand all of this old fear and emotion over to the Fire Red Ray to feel peace within yourself again. Hold this fiery love energy within your heart to help you heal the past. Now go to the steps in the far-right corner of this sacred space that leads to the next level. Climb the 12 steps as I count with you, 1, 2, 3, 4, 5, 6, 7, 8, 9, 10, 11, 12, you are now on the next level.

Level 4 - the consciousness of transition – we are joined by the light being Violet Ray – This level is made up of celestial layers between the third and fifth dimensions and is what we call the middle ground, the stepping-stone to the higher dimensions from the heavy 3D energy matrix level 3. Light being Violet Ray brings you a smoother flowing energy, offering new possibilities, capabilities, and clarity with its higher knowledge. Allow the Violet Ray energy to surround you so it can lead you away from karma, self-inflicted doubt, and negative feelings. Guiding you to wisdom, truth, love and aligning you with your incarnated soul. Imagine this beautiful Violet energy all around you, breathing in this light through your breath in and every pore of your body. Now go to the steps in the far-right corner of this sacred space that leads to the next level. Climb the 12 steps as I count with you, 1, 2, 3, 4, 5, 6, 7, 8, 9, 10, 11, 12, you are now on the next level.

Level 5 - the consciousness of unconditional love – we are joined by the light being Pink Ray– The light being Pink Ray energy brings you self-presence and trust to bring unconditional love into your sacred heart space. Allow Pink Ray to surround you with their love, breathing in this unconditional love that is present at all times in the universe and your soul. Take this energy deep within you connecting with your soul base. Feel this unconditional love and release any emotion if you feel the need to. Now go to the steps in the far-right corner of this sacred space that leads to the next level. Climb the 12 steps as I count with you, 1, 2, 3, 4, 5, 6, 7, 8, 9, 10, 11, 12, you are now on the next level.

Level 6 - the consciousness of creative ideas – we are joined by the light being Yellow Ray – The light being Yellow Ray brings a new doorway for you that leads to knowledge, wisdom and resolving the mysteries of the Earth through connecting to the halls of learning. Let this creative energy surround you as it helps you connect with and respect

Mother Earth and stay connected to the divine high source energy. Light being Yellow Ray also brings clear vision for clarity to the human mind bring in learning and communication so the telepathic process. Imagine this Yellow Ray energy entering your third eye and taking it to your pineal gland that sits under the crown chakra on top of your head. This is to help waken apart of your mind you are not using and building your link with the higher source of knowledge. Now go to the steps in the far-right corner of this sacred space that leads to the next level. Climb the 12 steps as I count with you, 1, 2, 3, 4, 5, 6, 7, 8, 9, 10, 11, 12, you are now on the next level.

Level 7 - the consciousness of harmonic sound – we are joined by the light being Azure Ray – Azure Ray brings to you in this level the harmonic sound energy, bringing in the energy of compassion, empathy, non-judgemental thoughts, patience, kindness, forgiveness, gratitude, and sincerity. Allow this beautiful energy to surround you breathing in the sound of creation that weaves together the structure of every cell of the universe and all we know. Imagine fine threads interweaving through the universe connected to everything, all creation held together by a divine vibration of harmonic sounds, and you are part of this amazing creation. Imagine this beautiful energy passing through your ears into your subconscious mind setting a higher frequency for your new ascension path of growth on Earth. Now go to the steps in the far-right corner of this sacred space that leads to the next level. Climb the 12 steps as I count with you, 1, 2, 3, 4, 5, 6, 7, 8, 9, 10, 11, 12, you are now on the next level.

Level 8 - the consciousness of new creation – we are joined by the light being Translucent Ray – The light being Translucent Ray brings you teachings of wisdom and philosophy. Allow this Translucent energy to surround you to prepare you for advance downloads and new knowledge. Remember every human is a teacher as you are, and we ask you share your experiences and knowledge we give you with others. Let this energy surround you and breathe in this beautiful energy for new creation on your life's path. Now go to the steps in the far-right corner of this sacred space that leads to the next level. Climb the 12 steps as I count with you, 1, 2, 3, 4, 5, 6, 7, 8, 9, 10, 11, 12, you are now on the next level.

Level 9 - the consciousness of manifestation – we are joined by the light being Astral Blue Ray - Astral Blue Ray brings you the multidimensional energy connection for the ethereal self. This is the level where the hierarchy of all form in the universe is established. As you progress though the Earth life and ascend, you can with careful thought process manifest from within a positive life. Allow this beautiful Astral Blue Ray energy to surround you and imagining it entering through your crown chakra traveling through every cell of your body. As you do this you are opening up the door of positive manifestation for yourself. Now go to the steps in the far-right corner of this sacred space that leads to the next level. Climb the 12 steps as I count with you, 1, 2, 3, 4, 5, 6, 7, 8, 9, 10, 11, 12, you are now on the next level.

Level 10 - the consciousness of truth – we are joined by the light being Indigo Ray– this level holds the living truth of all that was and will be and is the pure light from unconditional love that is within everything. Allow the Indigo Ray to surround you and feel this being's beautiful energy connect with your inner soul base and higher self. Now set the intension to allow your true spiritual life's mission to come forward on your life's path, always thinking and speaking your truth. Now go to the steps in the far-right corner of this sacred space that leads to the next level. Climb the 12 steps as I count with you, 1, 2, 3, 4, 5, 6, 7, 8, 9, 10, 11, 12, you are now on the next level.

Level 11 - the consciousness of the universe – we are joined by the light being Lilac Ray – this level holds the high divine energy where creation is triggered for all living things. The Lilac Ray brings the 12 principles of the universe, surround yourself with this beautiful powerful energy to allow them to retrigger memories held in your DNA and soul connection. With this activation we bring you the laws of oneness, vibration, relativity, rhythm, polarity, action, attraction, manifestation, karma, transmutation, gender, and intention. As the Lilac Ray surrounds you, embrace this unconditional love of the universe. You will feel this powerful energy in every cell of your being as we trigger this ancient knowledge. Now go to the steps in the far-right corner of this sacred space that leads to the next level. Climb the 12 steps as I count with you, 1, 2, 3, 4, 5, 6, 7, 8, 9, 10, 11, 12, you are now on the next level.

Level 12 - the consciousness of source - we are joined by the light being Silver Ray – This last level is the divine energy of creation and links us all in the light beings Silver Ray energy of love that passes through everything in the universe and the twelve-dimensional levels. The light being Silver Ray ensures the conscious source energy of the universe and sits within every living cell that exists. Allow the Silver Ray energy to enter your body's multidimensional field imaging it in every vibrational cell of your body, breathing in the unconditional love source of creation. Now hold this divine energy within your heart.

This final level now completes this beautiful pyramid ascension light meditation. In the centre of this twelfth level is a golden portal energy door go to the portal of golden energy and walk through it, you are now coming back into your three-dimensional energy space your room into full Earth consciousness. Take some deep breaths in, wriggle your toes and fingers. Ensure you have a drink of water to help ground you after this high vibration meditation. We advise you sit there for a few minutes so you can become fully aware of your personal space.

Thank you for participating in this wonder meditation, please share as part of your life's teaching to others. Love and blessings to you all.

Self-empowerment Meditation

This meditation has been channeled by us to help you acknowledge the powerful spiritual connection that is always within you. You are born into this 3D reality in a high energy vibrational frequency of unconditional love. You come with all the tools you need to survive this heaver 3D energy world called Earth. You have a powerful built-in inner connection some call the six sense. It is this empowerment of ancient energy and knowledge that is waiting to be unleashed. This meditation will help you tap into this to enhance your spiritual journey.

Meditation for Self-empowerment

Never meditate when driving or using machinery. Always be in a safe space where you can relax and not be disturbed and have a glass of water ready for after the meditation.

Now relax and shut your eyes and take your focus to your breathing, take in a deep breath, breathing in the love and light energy now surrounding you and release any worries, fears, and anxiety as you breath out. Take in another deep breath in, breathing in love and light energy. *(Do this a couple more times).*

Now imagine a golden energy ball the size of a tennis ball floating in front of your face. This beautiful powerful pulsating energy is your inner power from within you. You all use your five senses, sight, smell, taste, touch, and hearing to live your human life. These five senses combined are a powerful force on their own, as they act as your navigators to help you survive in the human world. The golden energy empowerment ball is your six sense that you are born with to connect to the higher divine energies. This energy helps you remember your life mission here on earth. This golden empowerment energy connects to the human body through the third eye, scared heart space and soul.

Focusing on this golden energy ball, I want you pull this

energy through you third eye that sits in the middle of your forehead. Feel the powerful force of this energy as it passes into your head. Now imagine this energy stopping under your crown chakra that sits on top of your head, where your deep conscious brain space and penal gland sits. Your high ascension being celestial guides connect with you telepathically using this part of your brain and your ethereal energy field. Your soul also is connected to this part of your brain to communicate with you.

See and feel this empowerment energy in your brain, now take this energy down through your neck to your sacred heart space that sits in the center of your breastbone. Now imagine within your body behind your sacred heart space a silver energy in an oval shape cylinder where your soul energy resides and is protected. The six-sense empowerment energy is now linking with your soul, pineal gland, deep conscious brain space and your third eye energy space. Feel this empowerment and visualise a silver thread that runs from your soul to the scared heart space, up through your deep conscious mind space and then passes through your crown chakra, connecting you to your higher self, the universe and the high divine energy source of unconditional love.

Place a hand on you sacred heart space and feel that connection within you. This is your own power that sits within you at all times. I will leave you for a short while with this connection. *(Three minutes of music gap here).*

I ask you now to TRUST the six sense and the powerful connection you have within yourself, the divine source and the universe. It brings you intuition, great strength and is your support system while here on Earth. Building this power from within will enhance your Earth life and if you are a lightworker your connection with spirit. Remember your thoughts are very powerful and a positive thought pattern and TRUST will keep you linked with this empowerment from within.

Focusing on your breath take a deep breath in, becoming more aware of your physical body. Take another deep breath in and wriggle your toes and fingers. Open your eyes and sit for a few minutes and then have some water.

Take time to reflect on your experience and learn to embrace this empowerment you were born with and use it for the good of self and humanity. Use this meditation when you feel disconnected from the source of the divine energy or a little bit lost on your Earth path. The meditation will always remind you of your power and life mission that's sits in your soul and the deep ancient ways that are recorded in your DNA consciousness.

Thank you for participating in this meditation, love, and blessings to you.

Peace of Mind Relaxation Meditation

It is key for a healthy mind and body to take time out from your busy life so you can relax, and this meditation is designed to help you do just that. This short meditation uses a mixture of breath technique and visualisation to help you achieve a state of relaxation. You can also use the breath focusing technique on your everyday lives to bring mindfulness and clarity of mind in stressful situations.

Meditation for Peace of mind relaxation

Never meditate when driving or using machinery. Always be in a safe space where you can relax and not be disturbed and have a glass of water ready for after the meditation as this will help ground you and refocus your mind.

Now relax and shut your eyes and take your focus to your breathing, take in a deep breath, breathing in the calming energy now surrounding you and release any worries, fears and anxiety as you breath out. Take in another a deep breath in, breathing in the calming energy.

Now concentrate your attention on your breath, your normal everyday breathing pattern. The breath will be centre stage of your awareness, just let your body breathe for itself as we do every day.

Take your awareness to the gentle flowing of the IN and OUT breath, notice how it feels travelling up and down your airways to your lungs. How does it feel in your nostrils, and then as your breath flows to your lungs?

Feel the breath leaving the body and re-entering.

Where do you feel the sensations? In the nostrils, mouth and stomach?

Relax and just ride the waves of your breathing moment by moment, with each breath.

Remind yourself of the attention you need to give this, concentrating on the breathing.

Can you smell the breath, is there any taste and are there sensations in your mouth?

Imagine the breath blowing out. Does it have colour, or is there any moisture?

If any past and present thoughts intrude, just gently and lovingly let the thoughts pass by, re-establishing focus on the breath.

Now expand your awareness to your whole body.

How does the breath feel as you breathe in and out? Your skin breathes, imagine the breath leaving every pore of your body, can you feel this? Take note of any sensations you pick up on.

Now take yourself back to focusing on the nostrils, the breath coming in and out of the body. Just rest on these feelings, being in the moment. I will now leave you focusing on your breath relaxing and enjoying your own personal space and the music for a short while. *(3 minutes)*

Feeling relaxed now focusing on your breath, take a deep breath in, becoming more aware of your physical body. Take another deep breath in and wriggle your toes and fingers. Open your eyes and sit for a few minutes and then have some water.

Use this meditation regularly to relax and help clear your mind of your busy daily thoughts. You will feel more relaxed and in tune with your mind and body.

Thank you for participating in this meditation, love, and blessings to you.

All meditations are available to download on https://www.etsy.com/uk/shop/BengalroseHealing

We offer a gift of a **fifty percent off discount code** on the six meditations you need for your Deep Core Healing. Please email sharon@bengalrose.co.uk for the code.

In this book, I have laid before you the pathway to self-healing and the power you hold to change your own future. Through the stories of two human life journeys, I have shown how uniquely designed you are and how a shift in perspective becomes the key to Deep Core Healing. I have also shared how this level of healing unfolds differently for every individual, honouring the sacred uniqueness of your soul's journey.

Within these pages, I have brought forward understandings of the Quantum Era, celestial beings and guides, energy communication, the higher self, the ethereal human essence, soul plan alignment, energy healing, Earth's awakening process, and much more. The guidance offered here provides foundational insights, stepping stones to help you navigate and anticipate the experiences that may arise throughout your spiritual healing journey.

My intention is that these words ignite your inner light, inspire transformation, and empower you to become a living representative of higher consciousness on Earth. To support you further, I have created a Deep Core Healing Workbook designed to assist and guide you through this process of inner restoration.

Trust that your celestial guides walk beside you every step of the way. Ask them to heal you, uplift you, and love you and you will begin to meet a renewed version of yourself: the true YOU.

About the Author

Sharon from Bengalrose Healing is a Light Worker Channeler, Author, Trance Communicator, Leader of spiritual and trance knowledge, and Spiritual Mentor based in South Wales, United Kingdom. Her book, **'Deep Core Healing'** is part of her collection of channelled books:

In paper back and on kindle
'The Art of Trance,
'I am a ginger haired girl with freckles'
'New Earth - The light over the horizon',
'Utopia', 'The Magic of Spirit',
'The Magic of Words',
'Past Lives',
'Step into the Mind of a Medium',
'Heavenly Guidance',
'The light within Atlantis',
Your Daily Spiritual Guidance Diary',
'The Celestial Guardians of Earth',
'A Path of Illumination',
'The Spiritual Tool Kit',
'A Journey Through Creation'.
Workbooks – Paper back only
'Awakening Your Spiritual Pathway',
'Spiritual Development for Beginners'
'Discover Your Starseed Origins'
'Deep Core Healing'

Sharon's books are available on Amazon worldwide and https://www.etsy.com/uk/shop/Bengalrose
Visit her website www.bengalrose.co.uk to find out more

about Sharon and what she offers.

MP3 and CD meditations available on
https://www.etsy.com/uk/shop/Bengalrose

Bengalrose is also on social media:
Facebook - www.facebook.com/SharonBengalroseHealing
YouTube - @sharonBarbourQTH-785
Instagram – BengalroseHealing
Linkedin - https://www.linkedin.com/in/sharon-milne-
barbour-53278a43/

Sharon also welcomes contact through email:
Sharon@bengalrose.co.uk

Quantum Trance Healing – QTH website is
www.quantumtrancehealing.co.uk
https://www.facebook.com/groups/523797893243609

We thank Amanda Bowden for her contribution to our book.

www.amandabowden.co.uk